A Practical Guide to Designing Phase II Trials in Oncology

STATISTICS IN PRACTICE

Series Advisors

Human and Biological Sciences
Stephen Senn
CRP-Santé, Luxembourg

Earth and Environmental Sciences
Marian Scott
University of Glasgow, UK

Industry, Commerce and Finance
Wolfgang Jank
University of Maryland, USA

Founding Editor
Vic Barnett
Nottingham Trent University, UK

Statistics in Practice is an important international series of texts which provide detailed coverage of statistical concepts, methods and worked case studies in specific fields of investigation and study.

With sound motivation and many worked practical examples, the books show in down-to-earth terms how to select and use an appropriate range of statistical techniques in a particular practical field within each title's special topic area.

The books provide statistical support for professionals and research workers across a range of employment fields and research environments. Subject areas covered include medicine and pharmaceutics; industry, finance and commerce; public services; the earth and environmental sciences; and so on.

The books also provide support to students studying statistical courses applied to the above areas. The demand for graduates to be equipped for the work environment has led to such courses becoming increasingly prevalent at universities and colleges.

It is our aim to present judiciously chosen and well-written workbooks to meet everyday practical needs. Feedback of views from readers will be most valuable to monitor the success of this aim.

A complete list of titles in this series appears at the end of the volume.

A Practical Guide to Designing Phase II Trials in Oncology

Sarah R. Brown

University of Leeds, UK

Walter M. Gregory

University of Leeds, UK

Chris Twelves

St James's University Hospital, Leeds, UK

Julia Brown

University of Leeds, UK

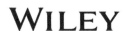

Library of Congress Cataloging-in-Publication Data

A practical guide to designing phase II trials in oncology / [edited by] Sarah R. Brown,
Walter M. Gregory, Christopher Twelves, Julia Brown.
    p. ; cm.
  Includes bibliographical references and index.
  ISBN 978-1-118-57090-6 (hardback)
  I. Brown, Sarah R., editor of compilation.   II. Gregory, Walter M., editor of compilation.
III. Twelves, Chris, editor of compilation.   IV. Brown, Julia (Julia M.), editor of compilation.
  [DNLM: 1. Clinical Trials, Phase II as Topic.   2. Antineoplastic Agents–therapeutic use.
3. Drug Evaluation–methods.   4. Neoplasms–drug therapy. QV 771.4]
  RC271.C5
  616.99′4061–dc23

                                   2013041156

A catalogue record for this book is available from the British Library.

ISBN: 978-1-118-57090-6

Set in 10/12pt Times by Aptara Inc., New Delhi, India

1   2014

To Austin, from Sarah, for your continued support and encouragement.

And to the many patients and their carers who take part in clinical trials, often at the most difficult of times, helping in the development of new and better treatments for people with cancer now and in the future.

Contents

6 Designs incorporating toxicity as a primary outcome   112

Sarah Brown

7 Designs evaluating targeted subgroups   131

Sarah Brown

Contributors

Sarah Brown Clinical Trials Research Unit, Leeds Institute of Clinical Trials Research, University of Leeds, UK.

———

This book was collectively written by Sarah Brown with contributions from:

Ornella Belvedere Department of Oncology, York Hospital, York, UK.

Julia Brown Clinical Trials Research Unit, Leeds Institute of Clinical Trials Research, University of Leeds, UK.

Marc Buyse International Drug Development Institute, Louvain-la-Neuve, Belgium.

John Chester Institute of Cancer and Genetics, School of Medicine, Cardiff University, and Honorary Consultant, Velindre Cancer Centre, Cardiff, UK.

Steven Green Novartis Pharma AG, Basel, Switzerland.

Walter Gregory Clinical Trials Research Unit, Leeds Institute of Clinical Trials Research, University of Leeds, UK.

Rick Kaplan Medical Research Council Clinical Trials Unit at University College London, University College London Hospital, and NIHR Cancer Research Network Coordinating Centre, UK.

William Mietlowski Novartis Pharma AG, Basel, Switzerland.

Mahesh Parmar Medical Research Council Clinical Trials Unit at University College London, and NIHR Cancer Research Network Coordinating Centre, UK.

Anthony Rossini Novartis Pharma AG, Basel, Switzerland.

Steve Schey Kings College, London, and Lead Myeloma Clinician, Kings College Hospital, London, UK.

Matthew Seymour Leeds Institute of Cancer and Pathology, University of Leeds, and NIHR Cancer Research Network, Leeds and National Cancer Research Institute, London, UK.

Chris Twelves Leeds Institute of Cancer and Pathology, University of Leeds, and St James's University Hospital, Leeds, UK.

Foreword I

The past two decades have seen an unprecedented expansion in the knowledge about the biological, immunological and molecular phenomena that drive malignancy. This knowledge has subsequently been translated into a large number of potential anti-cancer therapeutics and potential predictive or prognostic molecular markers that are under evaluation in clinical trials.

A key component of the oncology clinical trials development process is the bridge that must be crossed between the end of phase I evaluation of a drug, at which time information on its recommended dose, schedule, pharmacokinetic and pharmacodynamics effects in a small group of individuals is available, and the defini-tive randomised efficacy trial of that drug in the appropriately defined population of cancer patients.

This 'bridge' is provided by the phase II trial. Historically, phase II oncology stud-ies sought evidence of sufficient drug efficacy (based on objective tumour response in a specific cancer type) that large confirmatory phase III trials would be justified. Those not meeting the efficacy bar would not be pursued in further studies in that tumour type. In today's highly competitive environment, the phase II study has come under scrutiny – some have expressed the concern that too many 'promising' drugs emerging from phase II studies yield negative phase III results, that clinical trial end-points traditionally deployed in phase II may not be specific or sensitive enough for today's molecular-based agents to appropriately direct subsequent drug development decisions, that efficiency is lost if discrete phase II and phase III trials are designed and that much more should be learned about predictive or selection biomarkers before and during phase II to optimally guide phase III design.

Numerous papers and opinion pieces on these and other phase II–related topics have been published in the past decade. Thus this new book by Brown and colleagues: *A Practical Guide to Designing Phase II Trials in Oncology* is a welcome addition to the literature. This comprehensive and well-written guide takes a logical and step-by-step approach by reviewing and making recommendations on the key variables that must be considered in phase II oncology trials. Some of these include tailoring design components to the specific trial question, the approach to studies of single- and combination-agent trials, when and how randomised and adaptive designs might be deployed, patient selection and phase II trial endpoints. In addition, the book drills into issues that may be unique to designs in several specific malignancies such as non-small cell lung cancer, prostate cancer and myeloma. Throughout, examples are utilised as a means of providing context and guiding the reader.

What is clear is that the phase II oncology trial is not a singular or simple construct. There is no formula for its design that meets all potential needs. These trials the 'shape-shifters' of the cancer trial spectrum – how they are designed, the endpoints that are utilised, and the population enrolled depends on the agent and its associated biology, the type of cancer, the question the trial is intended to address and how those results are intended to guide future decisions. This comprehensive text provides much-needed practical information in this important area of clinical cancer research.

Elizabeth A. Eisenhauer, MD, FRCPC
Head, Department of Oncology
Queen's University
Kingston, ON, Canada

Foreword II

Twenty years ago, in the early 1990s, the term 'phase II trial design' was practically synonymous with the Simon optimal and MINIMAX two-stage trials (1989) – designs which have stood the test of time with their pragmatic trade-off between the need to stop a trial early for inefficacy if response rates were low and the likely overshoot of interim analysis points in small trials. The Gehan design was also widely used but many statisticians were wary of designs which focussed on estimation but did not have distinct success/failure rules which allowed error rates to be tightly specified.

The field of phase II trial design has expanded rapidly since these early days, particularly in oncology. Phase I trial design has also been extended over the years to go beyond mere dose finding and frequently includes an expansion phase at the chosen dose level which provides initial information on efficacy and pharmacodynamic predictors of response. Ideally this should enhance the relevance of the subsequent phase II trials.

This book presents a much-needed guide to contemporary phase II clinical trial design. Over the years trial endpoints have diversified to include the greater use of endpoints such as progression free survival that cater for treatments that may not cause tumour shrinkage and are thought to act by halting cancer cell growth rather than killing the cell (cytostatic rather than cytotoxic). Recognition of the inaccuracies inherent in designing trials on the basis of the expected response gleaned from historical data has also seen more focus on the use of randomisation and the incorporation of a control group. The increasing emphasis on stratified medicine, recognising the need to tailor treatments more closely to the biological characteristics of the individual patient's disease, has also led to phase II trials designed to address this need.

The recognition of the division between phase IIa trials designed to investigate efficacy and phase IIb trials, which focus on determining whether a phase III trial is worth undertaking, has also been welcome. The latter have increased in size and complexity in an effort to forestall the possibility of a negative phase III trial. It has been suggested that as many as two out of every three phase III oncology trials are negative – a situation which is of real concern, given that drug development is increasing in expense and comparatively few gain regulatory approval. It is reassuring to note the number of phase II/III designs that have been developed to closely link the development of phase II and phase III, but in some situations this is not possible.

The Simon Optimal Design (Simon 1989) is perhaps the seminal phase II single arm design, and it is salutary to see how frequently this design is used and has acted as a springboard for the development of other designs. It is frequently possible to add judiciously placed interim analyses to trials without increasing the number of patients or having an adverse effect on the error rates – a manoeuvre which is worth bearing in mind. For example, the two-stage Simon MINIMAX design, which minimises the number of patients needed to assess a binary endpoint, is frequently the same size as the one-stage exact design – on occasion, the MINIMAX design is even marginally smaller than the single-stage design! The MINIMAX design illustrates the point that an optional futility interim analysis can be built into a planned one-stage trial of a binary endpoint without increasing the number of patients or adversely affecting the error rates. Alternatively, note that a one-stage design can frequently be converted into a two-stage design by including a futility interim analysis at $N/2$ (here N is the fixed sample single-stage trial size or could be the number of events for a time-to-event endpoint). The trial would be stopped on the grounds of futility if the primary endpoint parameter did not exceed the value under the null hypothesis. This approach is seen in the design mentioned by Whitehead (2009, Section 4.2.1). A general boundary rule that I have also used is the $p \leq 0.001$ rule (Peto–Haybittle) and related to this are common-sense considerations that should not be overlooked. For example, if five or more responses in a 41-patient trial are needed to demonstrate efficacy, as soon as five responses have been observed the efficacy threshold for the trial has been passed, and it is clear a phase III trial will be recommended. If the toxicity profile is acceptable, the fact the efficacy criteria has been met should be disseminated so that planning for the follow-on phase III trial can commence.

This book will act as a valuable reference source in addition to giving sound practical guidance. The authors identify a number of areas that have not been explored; for example, no references were identified for randomised trials with a multinomial outcome measure (Section 4.1.3). Statisticians who read this book could perhaps ask themselves which neglected areas they think deserve the highest priority. As regards phase IIb designs, I would like to see a three-outcome version of the randomised Simon (2001) design (Section 4.1.4) based on progression-free survival.

Roger A'Hern
Senior Statistician
Clinical Trials and Statistics Unit
Institute of Cancer Research
Sutton, United Kingdom

Preface

Phase II trials are a key element of the drug development process in cancer, representing a transition from initial evaluation in relatively small phase I studies, not only focused on safety but also increasingly incorporating translational studies, to definitive assessment of efficacy often in large randomised phase III trials. Efficient design of these early phase trials is crucial to informed decision-making regarding the future of a drug's development. There are a number of textbooks available that discuss statistical issues in early phase clinical trials. These cover pharmacokinetics and pharmacodynamics studies, through to late phase II trials, and discuss issues around sample size calculation and methods of analysis. There are few, however, which focus specifically on phase II trials in cancer, and the many elements involved in their design. Given the large number and variety of phase II trial designs, often conceptually innovative, and involving multiple components, the purpose of this book is to provide practical guidance to researchers on appropriate phase II trial design in cancer.

This book provides an overview to clinical trial researchers of the steps involved in designing a phase II trial, from the initial discussions regarding the trial idea itself, through to identification of an appropriate phase II design. It is written as an aid to facilitate ongoing interaction between clinicians and statisticians throughout the design process, enabling informed decision-making and providing insight as to how information provided by clinicians feeds into the statistical design of a trial. The book acts both as a comprehensive summary resource of traditional and novel phase II trial designs and as a step-by-step approach to identifying suitable designs.

We wanted to provide a practical and structured approach to identifying appropriate statistical designs for trial-specific design criteria, considering both academic and industry perspectives. A comprehensive library of available phase II trial designs is included, and practical examples of how to use the book as a resource to design phase II trials in cancer are given. We have purposely omitted methodological detail associated with statistical designs for phase II trials, as well as discussion of analysis, that can be found elsewhere, including in the references for each of the designs listed in the library of designs.

The book begins with an introduction to phase II trials in cancer and their role within the drug development process. A structured thought process addressing the key elements associated with identifying appropriate phase II trial designs is introduced in Chapter 2, including therapeutic considerations, outcome measures and randomisation. Each of these elements is discussed in detail, describing the different stages of the thought process around which the guidance is centred. The purpose of this detailed information is to allow readers to narrow down the number of designs that are relevant to their trial-specific design criteria. A comprehensive library of phase II designs is presented in Chapters 3–7, categorised according to design criteria, and a brief summary of each trial design available is included.

Chapters 8–12 outline a series of practical examples of designing phase II trials in cancer, providing practical illustration from trial concept to using the library to select an appropriate trial design. The examples give a flavour of how one might apply the process described within the book, highlighting that there is no 'one size fits all' approach to trial design and that there are often many design solutions available to any one scenario. We hope the book will help researchers to shortlist their options in order to select an appropriate design to their specific setting, acknowledging other options that may be considered.

This book has been written predominantly by academic clinical trialists, involving both clinicians and statisticians. Many of the issues and considerations described from an academic point of view are, however, also relevant to trials sponsored by the pharmaceutical industry. The final chapter of this book describes the design of phase II trials in cancer from the industry perspective. The commercial perspective is described in detail, outlining the design processes for phase II trials according to specific strategic goals. This highlights both the similarities and differences in the approach to phase II trial design between academia and industry. In the academic setting there may be more focus on the phase II trial itself and less on the overall development programme of the drug, compared to industry where the trial is designed as part of a programme-oriented clinical development plan.

The book is written for both clinicians and statisticians involved in the design of phase II trials in cancer. Although some elements are written primarily with statisticians in mind, the discussion around key concepts of phase II trial design, as well as the practical examples, is accessible to scientists and clinicians involved in clinical trial design. For those new to early phase trial design, the book provides an introduction to the concepts behind informed decision-making in phase II trials, offering a unique and practical learning tool. For those familiar with phase II trial design, we hope the reader will benefit from exposure to new, less familiar trial designs, providing alternative options to those which they may have previously used. The book may also be used by postgraduate students enrolled on statistics courses including a clinical trial or medical module, providing a useful learning tool with core information on phase II trial design.

We hope that readers will benefit from the step-by-step approach described, as well as from the library of designs presented, enabling informed decision-making throughout the design process and focused guidance on designs that fit researchers' pre-specified criteria.

Finally, we would like to thank all our colleagues who have contributed to this book, for their advice and support.

1

Introduction

Sarah Brown, Julia Brown, Walter Gregory and Chris Twelves

Traditionally, cancer drug development can be defined by four clinical testing phases (Figure 1.1):

- Phase I is the first clinical test of a new drug after pre-clinical laboratory studies and is designed to assess the safety, toxicity and pharmacology of differing doses of a new drug. Typically such studies involve a limited number of patients and ask the question 'Is this drug safe?'

- Phase II studies are designed to answer the question 'Is this drug active, and is it worthy of further large-scale study?' They predominantly address the short-term activity of a new drug, as well as assessing further safety and toxicity. Typically sample sizes for phase II studies range from tens to low hundreds of patients.

- Phase III trials are often large-scale trials of hundreds, even thousands, of patients and are usually designed to formally evaluate whether a new drug is more effective in terms of efficacy or toxicity than current treatments. Here the focus generally is on long-term efficacy, with the aim of identifying practice-changing new drugs.

- Finally, phase IV studies are carried out once a drug is licensed or approved for a specific indication. Within the pharmaceutical industry setting, phase IV studies may be designed to collect long-term safety information; in the academic setting, phase IV trials may investigate the efficacy of a drug outside of its licensed indication.

A Practical Guide to Designing Phase II Trials in Oncology, First Edition.
Sarah R. Brown, Walter M. Gregory, Chris Twelves and Julia Brown.
© 2014 John Wiley & Sons, Ltd. Published 2014 by John Wiley & Sons, Ltd.

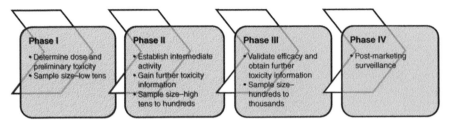

Figure 1.1   Four clinical phases of drug development.

Presented in this way drug development may appear to be a straight line pathway, but this is often not the case in practice, with much more time and money invested in large phase III trials than in other stages of development. Likewise, the boundaries between the different stages of drug development are increasingly blurred. For example, many phase I trials treat an expanded cohort of patients at the recommended phase II dose often at least in part to demonstrate proof of principle or seek evidence of activity. In recent years a wide range of new 'targeted' cancer therapies have emerged with well-defined mechanisms of action directed at specific molecular pathways relevant to tumour growth and often anticipated to be used in combination with other standard treatments. This contrasts with cytotoxic chemotherapy from which the traditional four phases of cancer drug development emerged. Nevertheless, phase II cancer trials retain their pivotal position between initial clinical testing and costly, time-consuming definitive efficacy studies.

The process from pre-clinical development to new drug approval typically takes up to 10 years and is estimated to cost hundreds of millions of dollars, although there is some uncertainty over the true costs (Collier 2009). Cytotoxic therapies, which lack a specific target and mechanism of action, often have a low therapeutic index, and historically have high rates of failure during drug development due to lack of efficacy and/or toxicity (Walker and Newell 2009). Although attrition rates for targeted cancer therapies appear lower than those of cytotoxic drugs, more drugs progress to expensive late stages of development before being abandoned in cancer than other therapeutic areas (DiMasi and Grabowski 2007). These worrying statistics have led to increased attention on clinical trial design, aiming to reduce the attrition rate and improve the efficiency of cancer drug development.

This book focuses on the high-risk transition between phase II and III clinical trials and provides a practical guide for researchers designing phase II clinical trials in cancer. There is a clear need for phase II trials that more accurately identify potentially effective therapies that should move rapidly to phase III trials; perhaps even more pressing is the need for earlier rejection of ineffective therapies before they enter phase III testing. On this basis we aim to provide researchers with a detailed background of the key elements associated with designing phase II trials in patients with cancer, a thought process for identifying appropriate statistical designs and a library of available phase II trial designs. The book is not intended to be proscriptive or didactic, but instead aims to facilitate and encourage an interactive approach by the clinical researcher and the statistician, leading to a more informed approach to designing phase II oncology trials.

1.1   The role of phase II trials in cancer

Phase II trials in cancer are primarily designed to assess the short-term activity of new treatments and the potential to move these treatments forward for evaluation of longer-term efficacy in large phase III studies. In this respect, the term 'activity' is used to describe the ability of an investigational treatment to produce an impact on a short-term or intermediate clinical outcome measure. We distinguish this from the term 'efficacy' which we use to describe the ability of an investigational treatment to produce a significant impact on a longer-term clinical outcome measure such as overall survival in a definitive phase III trial. Cancer phase II trials are therefore invariably conducted in the metastatic or neo-adjuvant settings, where measurable short-term assessments of activity are more easily obtained than in the adjuvant setting. We focus on phase II trials in cancer, where assessments of 'activity' are usually not immediate and cure not achievable. Nevertheless, many of the statistical designs available for phase II cancer trials, and concepts discussed, may be applied to other disease areas.

Phase II trials act as a screening tool to assess the potential efficacy of a new treatment. That broad description incorporates many different types of phase II trials including assessing not only traditional evidence of tumour response but also proof of concept of biological activity, selection between potential doses for further development, choosing between potential treatments for subsequent phase III testing and demonstration that the addition of a new agent to an established treatment appears to increase the activity of that treatment.

In 1982 Fleming stated that 'Commonly the central objective of phase II clinical trials is the assessment of the antitumor "therapeutic efficacy" of a specific treatment regimen' (Fleming 1982). More recently the objective of a phase II trial in an idealised pathway has been described to 'establish clinical activity and to roughly estimate clinical response rate in patients' (Machin and Campbell 2005). Others have taken this a step further to claim 'The objective of a phase II trial should not just be to demonstrate that a new therapy is active, but that it is sufficiently active to believe that it is likely to be successful in pivotal trials' (Stone et al. 2007a). A common feature of phase II trials is that their aim is not primarily to provide definitive evidence of treatment efficacy, as in a phase III study; rather, phase II trials aim to show that a treatment has sufficient activity to warrant further investigation.

The International Conference on Harmonisation (ICH) Guideline E8: General Considerations for Clinical Trials prefers to consider classification of study objectives rather than specific trial phases, since multiple phases of trials may incorporate similar objectives (ICH Expert Working Group 1997). The objectives associated with phase II trials in the ICH guidance are predominantly to explore the use of the treatment for its targeted indication; estimate or confirm dosage for subsequent studies; and provide a basis for confirmatory study design, endpoints and methodologies.

Additionally, however, ICH notes that phase II studies, on some occasions, may incorporate human pharmacology (assessing tolerance; defining or describing pharmacokinetics/pharmacodynamics; exploring drug metabolism and interactions; assessing activity) or therapeutic confirmation (demonstrating/confirming efficacy; establishing a safety profile; providing an adequate basis for assessing benefit/risk relationship for licensing; establishing a dose/response relationship).

These definitions have in common that oncology phase II trials act as an intermediate step between phase I testing on a limited number of patients to establish the safety of a new treatment and definitive phase III trials aiming to confirm the efficacy of a new treatment in a large number of patients. The specific aims of a phase II trial may, however, differ depending on the mechanism of action of the drug in question, the amount of information currently available on the drug and the setting in which it is being investigated (e.g. pharmaceutical industry vs. academia). Phase II trials can be broadly grouped into phase IIa and phase IIb trials. A phase IIa trial may be seen as seeking proof of concept in the sense of assessing activity of an investigational drug that has completed phase I development or may investigate multiple doses of a drug to determine the dose–response relationship. Phase IIa trials may be considered learning trials and be followed by a decision-making 'go/no-go' phase IIb trial to determine whether or not to proceed to phase III; phase IIb trials may include selection of a single treatment or dose from many and may include randomisation to a control arm.

Dose–response can be evaluated throughout the early stages of drug development, including phase II, but this book does not specifically address studies where this is the primary aim. Many designs are available to assess the dose–response relationship, perhaps the simplest and most common being the randomised parallel dose–response design incorporating a control arm and at least two differing dose levels. Cytotoxics are usually given at the highest feasible dose, but investigating dose–response relationships may be important with targeted agents that are not necessarily best given at the maximum possible dose. Such trials serve a number of objectives including the confirmation of efficacy; the estimation of an appropriate dose; the identification of optimal strategies for individual dose adjustments; the investigation of the shape and location of the dose–response curve; and the determination of a maximal dose beyond which additional benefit would be unlikely to occur.

Considerations around choice of starting dose, study design and regulatory issues in obtaining dose–response information are provided in the ICH Guideline E4: Dose Response Information to Support Drug Registration (ICH Expert Working Group 1994). Such considerations are, however, outwith the remit of this book, which focuses on phase II trials designed to assess activity of single-agent or combination therapies or those designed to select the most active of multiple therapies. We do, however, discuss phase II selection designs to identify the most active dose from a number of pre-specified doses rather than specific issues around evaluating dose–response relationships.

There are often significant differences between trials conducted within the pharmaceutical industry and those conducted within academia. Such differences are predominantly associated with the approach to designing phase II trials, within a portfolio of research, and decision-making around the future development of a compound or drug. Consequently, the way in which clinical trials are designed, particularly in the early phase setting, will likely differ between the two environments. For example, in the academic setting, regardless of the specific aim of the phase II trial (e.g. proof of concept, go/no-go), decision criteria are pre-specified to correspond with the primary aim of the trial and form the criteria on which decision-making and conclusions of the trial are based. Within the pharmaceutical industry the same pre-defined study aims and objectives apply; however, decision-making may be complicated by additional factors external to the phase II trial itself, such as the presence of competitor compounds, patent life or company strategy. There is inherent pressure within the pharmaceutical industry to achieve timely regulatory approval and a license indication for a new drug. This does not apply in the same way within the academic setting where, by the time a drug reaches phase II testing, it may have been through considerable testing within the pharmaceutical setting and perhaps be already licensed in alternative disease areas or in differing combinations or schedules. There are, however, initiatives to facilitate increased academic/pharmaceutical collaboration in the early stages of drug development. Thus, more academic phase II trials may be conducted using novel agents with only limited clinical data available, so thorough discussion of the aims and design of these trials becomes even more pertinent. A detailed insight into the industry approach to the design of phase II trials within a developing drug portfolio is provided in Chapter 13. By contrast, the remainder of this book, including terminology and practical examples of designing phase II trials, draws its focus from the academic setting.

1.2   The importance of appropriate phase II trial design

Design of phase II trials is a key aspect of the drug development process. Poor design may lead to increased probabilities of a false-positive phase II trial resulting in unnecessary investment in an unsuccessful phase III trial; or a false-negative phase II resulting in the rejection of a potentially effective treatment. There is a pressing need for phase II trials to more accurately identify those cancer therapies that will ultimately be successful in phase III studies and to allow earlier rejection of ineffective therapies before undertaking costly and time-consuming phase III trials.

As the development of new cancer drugs moves further away from conventional cytotoxics and more into targeted therapies, the challenges and opportunities in phase II trial design are ever greater. The choice of phase II design includes not only statistical considerations, but also decisions regarding the aims of the trial, whether or not to include randomisation, the choice of endpoints and the size of treatment effects to be targeted. Each of these elements is critical to ensure the phase II trial is designed and conducted efficiently and that the results of the trial may be used to make robust, informed decisions regarding future research.

Some researchers have suggested moving directly from phase I to phase III in the drug development process, on the basis that survival benefit in phase III trials may be observed in the absence of improved response rates therefore rendering phase II irrelevant (Booth et al. 2008). The potential perils of this approach are demonstrated by the INTACT1 and INTACT2 trials of gefitinib in chemotherapy-naïve advanced non-small cell lung cancer (NSCLC) patients (Giaccone et al. 2004; Herbst et al. 2004). Phase I trials of gefitinib in combination with chemotherapy had shown acceptable tolerability and gefitinib as monotherapy was active in phase II NSCLC trials; however, phase II trials of gefitinib in combination with chemotherapy were not performed. Subsequently, these two phase III NSCLC trials in over 2000 patients failed to show improved efficacy with the addition of gefitinib to cisplatin-based chemotherapy (Giaccone et al. 2004; Herbst et al. 2004). A conventional, single-arm NSCLC trial of gefitinib in combination with chemotherapy may have avoided the subsequent negative phase III trials. This experience highlights the importance of designing and conducting appropriately designed and potentially novel phase II trials prior to embarking on large-scale phase III trials.

1.3 Current use of phase II designs

Several systematic reviews have considered current use of designs in published phase II trials in cancer (Lee and Feng 2005; Mariani and Marubini 2000; Perrone et al. 2003). Common approaches to trial design included single-arm studies with objective response as the primary efficacy endpoint, utilising Simon's two-staged hypothesis testing methods (Simon 1989), and randomised trials based on single-arm designs embedded in a randomised setting (Lee and Feng 2005). All highlighted a distinct lack of detail regarding an identifiable statistical design, and design characteristics, as a marked weakness of many published phase II studies, raising the possibility that low quality may bias study findings. Also striking is the consistent use of a limited number of the same phase II study designs, emphasising the need for better understanding of alternative statistical designs. A key recommendation from these reviews is better communication between statisticians and clinical trialists to increase the use of newer statistical designs. Likewise, the need for 'the development of practical designs with good statistical properties and easily accessible computing tools with friendly user interface' (Lee and Feng 2005) is recognised as essential so statisticians can implement these new designs.

In 2009 the *Journal of Clinical Oncology* (*JCO*) published an editorial making recommendations for the types of phase II trials that they would consider for publication (Cannistra 2009). The differing aims of phase II trials according to the nature of the treatment under investigation were identified, with discussion as to the likely priority given to each trial design. The specific categories and outcomes of phase II trials were

- single-arm phase II studies that represent the first evidence of activity of a new drug class;

- phase II studies of novel agents that not only confirm a class effect, but also provide evidence of extraordinary and unanticipated activity compared to prior agents in the same class;

- phase II studies of an agent or regimen with prior promise (based on previous reports of clinical activity), but that are convincingly negative when studied more rigorously;

- phase II studies of a single-agent or combination that convincingly demonstrate a new, serious and unanticipated toxicity signal, despite being a rational and potentially active regimen;

- phase II studies with biomarker correlates that validate mechanism of action, provide convincing insight into novel predictive markers or permit enrichment of patients most likely to benefit from a novel agent;

- randomised phase II studies such as randomised selection, randomised comparison and randomised discontinuation designs.

The consistent use of single-arm, two-stage, response-driven designs as depicted in the systematic reviews described previously would not optimally cover the majority of these trial scenarios. The categories listed above were intended to provide authors with guidance as to the types of phase II trials most relevant to informing the design of subsequent phase III trials. Such recommendations highlight the need for awareness of the many components contributing to the design of phase II trials and the importance of making informed decisions to achieve the objectives of a trial and ensure the results are robust and interpretable.

1.4   Identifying appropriate phase II trial designs

This book aims to provide guidance to both the clinical researcher and statistician on each of the key elements of phase II trial design, enabling an understanding of how they inform the overall design process. Recommendations published by the Clinical Trial Design Task Force of the National Cancer Institute Investigational Drug Steering Committee (Seymour et al. 2010) and by the Methodology for the Development of Innovative Cancer Therapies (MDICT) Task Force (Booth et al. 2008) provide guidance on current best practice for individual aspects of early clinical trial design. General discussion of choice of endpoints and use of randomisation is given for the differing settings of monotherapy and combination therapy trials (Seymour et al. 2010), as well as in the specific context of targeted therapies (Booth et al. 2008), and discussion on reporting of phase II trials is also provided. Neither set of recommendations, however, provides detailed guidance on the statistical design categories available for phase II trials. Here we aim to guide researchers in a step-by-step manner through the thought process associated with each element of phase II design, from initial trial concept to the identification of an appropriate statistical design. With detailed discussion on each of the elements we aim to provide researchers with a thorough understanding of the overall process and each of the stages involved, therefore providing a more informed approach.

Central to this approach is an overall thought process, presented in detail in Chapter 2 and outlined briefly below. The approach consists of three stages, highlighting eight key elements associated with identifying an appropriate phase II trial design:

- Stage 1 – Trial questions:

  o Therapeutic considerations

  o Primary intention of trial

  o Number of experimental treatment arms

  o Primary outcome of interest

- Stage 2 – Design components:

  o Outcome measure and distribution

  o Randomisation

  o Design category

- Stage 3 – Practicalities:

  o Practical considerations

Each of these elements is discussed in detail in Chapter 2, and practical examples of using this approach to design phase II cancer trials are provided in Chapters 8–12. These elements were identified as being essential to the design of phase II trials in cancer through a comprehensive literature review of available statistical methodology for phase II trials (Brown et al. 2011). The thought process itself is iterative, such that information obtained during discussion of each element may feed into and inform later elements of the design. The starting point of any trial design should, however, be a discussion between the clinical researcher and the statistician that primarily concerns clinical factors relating to the specific treatment(s) under investigation (Stage 1). Continued interaction between the clinician and the statistician is essential throughout the design process.

Using the detail provided in Chapter 2, each of the elements is addressed in turn and iteratively. Decisions made throughout the process enable the statistician to narrow down the specific statistical designs appropriate to the pre-specified criteria. These statistical designs are provided in Chapters 3–7, a library resource of statistical designs, as introduced here. Each design is categorised to enable efficient navigation and identification of appropriate designs. Designs are laid out taking into account

- The use of randomisation including

  o Single-arm designs, arranged by design category and outcome measure – Chapter 3 o Randomised designs, arranged by design category and outcome measure – Chapter 4

o Treatment selection designs, arranged by inclusion of a control arm, design category and outcome measure – Chapter 5

- The focus on both activity and toxicity, or toxicity alone, as the primary outcome of interest – Chapter 6

- The evaluation of treatment activity in targeted subgroups – Chapter 7

Within each of Chapters 3–5, where there is no identified literature for specific design category and outcome measure combinations, this is highlighted within the relevant subsection. For example, there were no references identified discussing single-arm trial designs specifically focused on continuous outcome measures, therefore this subsection is included to highlight this to the reader. For Chapters 6 and 7, only those specific design category and outcome measure combinations for which references have been identified are listed, since generally there are fewer designs focused on activity and toxicity and targeted subgroups.

In the majority of cases there will be more than one statistical design that suits the pre-specified trial parameters determined via the thought process. In such cases, the final stage in the thought process, that of practical considerations, may allow a choice to be made between the alternatives. On the other hand, that choice may be based on previous experience or assessment of various trial scenarios by mathematical modelling or simulation. Further detail on choosing between multiple designs is provided in Chapter 2.

1.5   Potential trial designs

The statistical designs summarised in Chapters 3–7 were identified from a comprehensive literature review of phase II statistical design methodology conducted in January 2008 and updated in January 2010 (Brown et al. 2011). Individual designs were specifically assessed to determine their ease of implementation. Designs were defined as not easy to implement if

- the data required to enable implementation were not likely to be available;

- there was no sample size justification rendering the design difficult or impossible to interpret;

- criteria were not specified for the study being positive or negative as this makes the trial of little if any use in taking a new treatment forward;

- each patient needed to be assessed prior to the next patient being recruited, as this will usually be prohibitively restrictive in a phase II cancer trial; and

- the necessary statistical softwares were not detailed as being available and/or insufficient detail was provided to enable implementation.

While this assessment of ease of implementation is inherently subjective, these criteria reflect the practicalities of design implementation.

Applying the above criteria, those designs classed as being easy to implement are included in Chapters 3–7. This amounts to over 100 statistical designs, ranging from Gehan's original two-stage design published in 1961 (Gehan 1961) to complex multi-arm, multi-stage designs of more recent years. Mariani and Marubini highlighted researchers' preferences for single-arm, two-stage designs (Mariani and Marubini 2000); there are, however, a wealth of alternative designs available, ranging from adaptations of Simon's original two-stage design to incorporate adjustments for over-/under-recruitment, to randomised trials with formal hypothesis testing between experimental and control arms. The intention of this book is to present researchers with the designs available to them for their specific trial, rather than to recommend one design over another. In doing so we incorporate the well-established designs of Gehan (1961), Fleming (1982) and Simon (1989), as well as bringing lesser known designs to the attention of researchers, allowing the user to make informed choices regarding trial design. A brief overview of each design identified is presented; however, the technical detail of each design is omitted and may be further evaluated by considering the complete references, as appropriate.

With the continued development of targeted therapies in cancer, and a drive towards personalised medicine, the role of biomarkers within phase II trials is an important area for discussion. Where known biomarkers are available to identify selected patient populations most likely to benefit from an intervention, phase II trials may be designed as enrichment trials, whereby only biomarker-positive patients are included. In these cases, any of the statistical designs listed within Chapters 3–6 may be appropriate, focusing solely on the target population. Alternatively, when selected populations are perhaps less well validated, biomarker-stratified designs may be considered. Here both biomarker-positive and biomarker-negative subgroups are explored within a trial, ensuring adequate numbers of patients within each cohort to potentially detect differing treatment effect sizes. Such designs are listed within Chapter 7. A more detailed discussion of the incorporation of biomarkers within phase II trials in cancer is provided in Chapter 2. There have, however, been a number of recently published articles in this area that may not be included in the library of available statistical designs since they post-date the updated systematic review on which the library is based. Where the incorporation of biomarkers is of particular relevance to a trial design, the researcher may use the thought process described within this book and should consider not only any appropriate designs identified in Chapters 3–7, but also additional, more recent, designs specifically intended for trials incorporating biomarkers.

1.6   Using the guidance to design your trial

We present a thought process for the design of phase II trials in cancer, introduced briefly in Section 1.4, addressing the key elements associated with identifying an appropriate trial design; each of these elements is discussed in detail in Chapter 2.

The information in Chapter 2 will allow researchers to narrow down the number of appropriate designs for their trial and then navigate to the relevant designs in Chapters 3–7, where a brief summary of each trial design is provided. The statistical theory underpinning the designs detailed is published elsewhere (Mariani and Marubini 1996; Machin et al. 2008; Machin and Campbell 2005), as well as in the individual papers referenced.

This process is illustrated in Chapters 8–12 by a series of practical, real-life examples of designing phase II trials in cancer following the thought process and library of statistical designs. The examples are intended merely as pragmatic illustrations of how one might apply the process described within the book; they should not be taken as sole solutions to trial design under the particular settings presented. It is acknowledged that there may be a number of appropriate designs available, and exploration of various possibilities is encouraged. Examples are presented in the setting of head and neck cancer, lung cancer, prostate cancer, myeloma and colorectal cancer. Each example gives differing trial design scenarios highlighting various common issues encountered when designing phase II trials in cancer. These examples demonstrate the types of discussions expected between statisticians and clinicians in order to extract the necessary information to design a phase II trial. They also provide practical advice regarding how choice of design may be made when several designs fit the trial-specific requirements.

2

Key points for consideration

Sarah Brown, Julia Brown, Marc Buyse, Walter Gregory, Mahesh Parmar and Chris Twelves

Designing a phase II trial requires ongoing discussion between the clinician, statistician and other members of the trial team, so the design can evolve on the basis of information specific to each trial. Central to the approach of identifying an optimal phase II trial design is the thought process introduced in Chapter 1, and presented diagrammatically in Figure 2.1. The process provides an overview of the key stages and elements for consideration during the phase II trial design process. Each of these elements should be worked through in turn in an iterative manner as information derived at earlier stages feeds in to design choices and decisions in the latter stages and consideration of alternative designs.

The thought process is made up of three stages:

- Stage 1 – Trial questions. This stage elicits information predominantly relating to the trial itself in relation to the treatment under investigation, the primary intention of the trial, number of arms and primary outcome of interest.

- Stage 2 – Design components. The information from the first stage feeds into the discussions relating to design components considering the outcome measure, randomisation (or not) and category of design, enabling attention to be focused on the specific statistical designs relevant to the trial.

- Stage 3 – Practicalities. Finally, practical considerations may inform which, from a number of candidate trial designs, is the one best suited to a particular situation.

A Practical Guide to Designing Phase II Trials in Oncology, First Edition.
Sarah R. Brown, Walter M. Gregory, Chris Twelves and Julia Brown.
© 2014 John Wiley & Sons, Ltd. Published 2014 by John Wiley & Sons, Ltd.

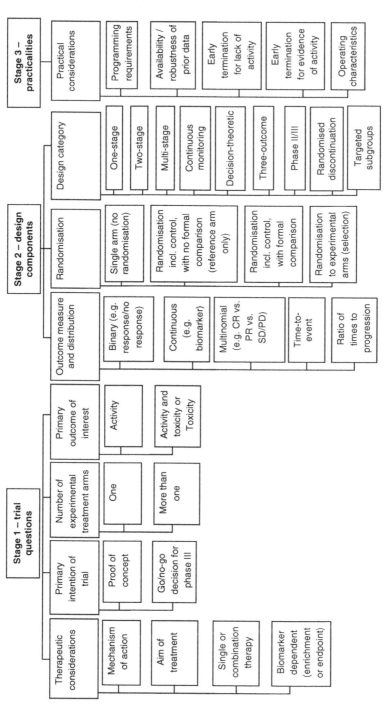

Figure 2.1 Thought process for identifying phase II trial designs.

This chapter works through each of the stages and components of Figure 2.1.

2.1   Stage 1 – Trial questions

2.1.1   Therapeutic considerations

The choice of trial design depends not only on statistical considerations, but more importantly on the clinical factors relating to the treatment(s) and/or disease under investigation. Discussion of these therapeutic considerations is essential to inform decisions to be made later in the thought process. At the first meeting between the clinician and statistician, discussion of the following points will provide an overview of the setting of the trial and the specific therapeutic issues to be incorporated into the trial design.

2.1.1.1   Mechanism of action

An important question to ask when beginning the trial design process is 'how does this treatment work?' The term 'cytotoxic' may be used to describe chemothera-peutic agents, where tumour shrinkage or response is widely accepted as reflecting anti-cancer activity. Many new cancer therapies are, however, targeted at specific molecular pathways relevant to tumour growth, apoptosis (programmed cell death) or angiogenesis (new blood vessel formation). Such 'targeted therapies', including tyrosine kinase inhibitors, monoclonal antibody therapies and immunotherapeutic agents, may be 'cytostatic'. Here, a change in tumour volume may not be the expected outcome: in such cases, tumour stabilisation or delay in tumour progression may be a more anticipated outcome.

The mechanism of action of the agent under investigation will inform many subsequent decisions, including the choice of outcome measure and whether or not the trial should be randomised.

2.1.1.2   Aim of treatment

The aim of the treatment under investigation should be considered both in the context of its mechanism of action and the specific population of patients in which the treatment is being considered.

It is important to consider the ultimate aim of treatment, which would inform the outcome measures in future phase III studies, and how this relates to shorter term aims that can be incorporated into phase II trials. For example, in a population of patients with a relatively long median progression-free survival (PFS) and overall survival (OS), the aim of a phase III trial may be to prolong further PFS and/or OS. These would, however, be unrealistic short-term outcomes for a phase II trial; tumour response, which may reflect PFS or OS, can be an appropriate shrinkage aim in a phase II trial. By contrast, where the prognosis is less good PFS may provide a realistic short-term outcome in phase II.

It is essential to consider how the longer term and shorter term aims of treatment are related, to ensure an appropriate intermediate outcome measure is chosen in phase II that provides a robust assessment of potential efficacy in subsequent phase III trials.

2.1.1.3   Single or combination therapy

It is important to ascertain whether the treatment under investigation will be given as a single agent or in combination with another novel or established intervention. This distinction can inform the decision as to whether or not randomisation should be incorporated. Where an investigational agent, be it a conventional cytotoxic or a targeted agent, is used in combination with another active treatment it can be very difficult to distinguish the effect of the investigational agent from that of the standard partner therapy; this distinction can be made easier by incorporating randomisation (see Section 2.2.2 for further discussion).

Similarly, the assessment of toxicity for combination treatments should also be addressed. Where the addition of an investigational therapy is expected to increase both activity *and* toxicity to a potentially significant degree, dual primary endpoints may be considered to assess the 'trade-off' between greater activity and increased toxicity (see Section 2.1.4 for further discussion).

2.1.1.4   Biomarker dependent

Biomarkers are an increasingly important part of clinical trials. They can be defined as 'a characteristic that is objectively measured and evaluated as an indicator of normal biological processes, pathogenic processes, or pharmacologic responses to a therapeutic intervention' (Atkinson et al. 2001).

Biomarkers may be considered in the design of phase II trials in two ways. First, a biomarker may serve as an outcome measure. The biomarker may be an intermediate (primary) endpoint in a phase II trial provided it reflects the activity of a treatment and is associated with efficacy; this may form the basis for a stop/go decision regarding a subsequent phase III trial. Decisions regarding the use of biomarkers as primary outcome measures will feed into the decision regarding use of randomisation, considering whether any historical data exist for the biomarker with the standard treatment and the reliability of such data. Where a change in a biomarker reflects the biological activity of an agent, but is not predictive of the natural history of the disease, this alone may be an appropriate endpoint for a proof of concept phase II trial; in such cases a second, go/no-go phase IIb trial may be required to assess the impact of the treatment on the cancer prior to a decision on proceeding to a phase III trial. The use of biomarkers as outcome measures is discussed further in Section 2.2.1.

Second, in the era of targeted therapies a molecular characteristic of the tumour that is relevant to the mechanism of action of the treatment under investigation may serve as a biomarker to define a specific subgroup of patients in whom an intervention is anticipated to be effective. This has been done especially successfully in studies of small molecules and monoclonal antibodies targeting HER-2 and related cell surface receptors (Piccart-Gebhart et al. 2005; Slamon et al. 2001). The potential for a biomarker to identify a subpopulation of patients may, however, only become apparent after phase III investigation, as in the case of the monoclonal antibody cetuximab in colon cancer where efficacy is limited to patients with no mutation in the *KRAS* oncogene (Bokemeyer et al. 2009; Tol et al. 2009; Van Cutsem et al. 2009). Where available, using a biomarker to enrich the population in a phase II trial in this way can increase the likelihood of anti-tumour activity being identified, and thus speed up drug development. By definition, when using a biomarker for population enrichment, the resulting phase II population is not representative of the general population. Interpreting outcomes in the enriched population may, therefore, be more challenging as historical control data may be unreliable; randomisation incorporating a control arm should be considered in such situations.

There are, however, potential risks with an over-reliance on biomarkers in phase II trials. If the mode of action of a novel therapy has been incorrectly characterised, the biomarker chosen for enrichment may be inappropriate and could lead to a false-negative phase II trial because the wrong patient population has been treated. Likewise, if a biomarker used to demonstrate proof of principle of biological activity does not accurately reflect the clinically relevant mode of action, the outcome of a phase II trial may be misleading. When a biomarker is the primary endpoint for a trial or used to enrich the patient population of patients it is vital that the biomarker be adequately validated. Where there is insufficient evidence that a biomarker reliably reflects biological activity or identifies an optimal patient group, measurement of the biomarker in an unselected phase II trial population may be appropriate as a hypothesis-generating exercise for future studies.

Approaches to trial design that incorporates biomarker stratification are discussed further in Section 2.2.3.

2.1.2   Primary intention of trial

In this context, we define the 'intention' of a trial not as the specific research question but in the wider sense of classifying trials into two categories:

- proof of concept, be that biological or therapeutic, or phase IIa;

- go/no-go decision for further evaluation in a phase III trial, or phase IIb.

A proof of concept, or phase IIa, trial may be undertaken after completing a phase I trial to screen the investigational treatment for initial evidence of activity. This may then be followed by a go/no-go phase IIb trial to determine whether a phase III trial is justified. Running two sequential phase II trials may, in some cases, be inefficient. The Clinical Trial Design Task Force of the National Cancer Institute Investigational Drug Steering Committee proposed that, where appropriate, proof of concept may be embedded in a single go/no-go trial (Seymour et al. 2010).

A model that is increasingly relevant to the development of targeted anti-cancer agents is to incorporate proof of concept translational imaging and/or molecular/biomarker studies within the expanded cohort of patients treated at the recommended phase II dose in a phase I trial. Where clear proof of concept can be demonstrated in this way, there is a blurring of the conventional divide between phase I and IIa studies but the need remains for a subsequent phase IIb trial with the intention of making a formal decision regarding further evaluation in a phase III trial.

While this specific point for consideration is not used to group the trial designs given in Chapters 3–7, it is important in considering issues such as primary outcome measures and the use of randomisation. Where a trial is designed as a proof of concept study alone, it may be appropriate to conduct a single-arm trial to obtain an estimate of the potential activity of a treatment to within an acceptable degree of accuracy. Short-term clinical or biomarker outcomes may be appropriate to give a preliminary assessment of activity prior to embarking on a larger scale phase IIb study. Where the aim of the phase II trial is to determine whether or not to continue evaluation of a treatment within a large-scale phase III trial, the ability to make formal comparisons between experimental and standard treatments may be more appropriate, to be more confident of that decision to proceed or not. Similarly, in phase IIb trials outcome measures known to be strongly associated with the primary phase III outcome measure are desirable for robust decision-making. Further discussion on the choice of outcome measures and the use of randomisation is given in Sections 2.2.1 and 2.2.2, respectively.

2.1.3   Number of experimental treatment arms

Whereas historically phase II cancer trials invariably had a single-arm, an increasing number now comprise multiple arms, one of which is often a 'control' standard treatment arm. The most common randomised phase II cancer trial designs have a single experimental arm with a control arm so the activity seen in the experimental arm can be compared formally or informally with that seen in the control arm. Randomisation may be appropriate where historical data on the outcome measure are unreliable or when a novel agent is being added to an effective standard therapy (see Section 2.2.2 for discussion).

Where multiple experimental treatments are available, or a single treatment that may be effective using different doses or schedules, a phase II trial may be designed to select which, if any, of these options should be taken forward for phase III evaluation. Randomisation can also be used to evaluate multiple treatment strategies such as the sequence of first- and second-line treatments. In these settings assessment of activity of each individual novel treatment, based on pre-specified minimal levels of activity, can be assessed using treatment selection designs which are described in Chapter 5.

Where multiple treatments are being investigated in a single phase II trial, with each single treatment in a different subgroup of patients (e.g. treatment A in biomarker-X-positive patients, and treatment B in biomarker-X-negative patients), this should *not* be considered as a treatment selection trial since only one experimental treatment is being investigated within each subgroup. For the purposes of trial design, such trials fall under the 'single experimental arm' category. Further discussion regarding trials of subgroups of patients is provided in Section 2.2.3.

2.1.4   Primary outcome of interest

The primary outcome of interest will depend on the existing evidence base and/or stage of development of the treatment under investigation, its mechanism of action and potential toxicity. Thus, information obtained from discussion of the therapeutic considerations of the treatment is important in deciding the primary focus of the trial, as well as incorporating data from previous studies of the same, or similar, treatments. At this stage, for the purpose of categorising trial designs, the primary outcome of interest is categorised as being either activity alone, or both activity and toxicity. Designs are also available that address a third option, of considering toxicity alone as the primary outcome measure in a phase II trial. These designs are incorporated with those assessing both activity and toxicity and are described in Chapter 6. Discussion regarding the specific primary clinical outcome measure is given in Section 2.2.1.

2.1.4.1   Activity

Where the toxicity of the investigational treatment is believed to be modest in the context of phase II decision-making or the toxicity of agents in the same class is well known, the *primary* phase II trial outcome measure will usually be anti-tumour activity, with toxicity included amongst the secondary outcome measures.

2.1.4.2   Activity and toxicity (or toxicity alone)

If the toxicity profile of the investigational treatment, be it a single-agent or combination therapy, is of particular concern, the activity and toxicity of the treatment may be considered as joint primary outcome measures, such that the investigational treatment must show both promising activity and an acceptable level of toxicity to warrant further evaluation. Such designs allow incorporation of trade-offs between pre-specified levels of increased activity and increased toxicity, to determine the acceptability of a new treatment with respect to further evaluation in a phase III trial.

2.2   Stage 2 – Design components

2.2.1   Outcome measure and distribution

Emerging cancer treatments have many differing modes of action, which should be reflected in the choice of outcome measures used to assess their activity. While tumour response according to Response Evaluation Criteria in Solid Tumours (RECIST) (Eisenhauer et al. 2009) has historically been the most widely used primary outcome measure, non-binary definitions or volumetric measures of response, measures of time to an event such as disease progression or continuous markers such as biomarkers may be more relevant when evaluating the activity of targeted or cytostatic agents (Adjei et al. 2009; Booth et al. 2008; Dhani et al. 2009; Karrison et al. 2007; McShane et al. 2009).

    When choosing between the many possible primary outcome measures for a phase II trial the key points to consider include the expected mechanism of action of the intervention under evaluation, the aim of treatment in the current population of patients, whether there are any biomarker outcome measures available, the stage of assessment in the drug development pathway (i.e. phase IIa or IIb) and the strength of the association between the proposed phase II outcome measure and the primary outcome measure that would be used in future phase III trials. The chosen outcome measure should also be robust with respect to external factors such as investigator bias and patient and/or data availability.

The primary outcome measure of a phase II trial should be chosen on the basis that if a treatment effect is observed, this provides sufficient evidence that a treatment effect on the phase III primary outcome is likely to be seen. The use of surrogate endpoints has been investigated in a number of disease areas, including breast (Burzykowski et al. 2008), colorectal (Piedbois and Buyse 2008) and head and neck cancer (Michiels et al. 2009). While the outcome measures used in phase II trials do not need to fulfil formal surrogacy criteria (Buyse et al. 2000) evidence of correlation between the phase II and III outcome measures is important to ensure reliability in decision-making at the end of a phase II trial.

The choice of primary outcome measures for a phase II trial reflects the outcome distribution. This section outlines the various options used to categorise phase II trial designs within Chapters 3–7, according to the distribution of the chosen primary outcome measure (as described in Chapter 1).

2.2.1.1   Binary

Response is usually evaluated via a continuous outcome measure, that is, the percentage change in tumour size. This is, however, typically dichotomised as 'response' versus 'no response' following RECIST criteria (Eisenhauer et al. 2009). Such binary outcomes, categorised as 'yes' or 'no', may be used for any measure that can be reduced to a dichotomous outcome including toxicity or change in a biomarker. Other outcome measures that may be expressed as continuous, such as time to disease progression, are frequently dichotomised to reflect an event rate, such as progression at a fixed time point.

In phase II studies of cytotoxic chemotherapy the biological rationale for response as an indicator of anti-cancer activity is based in part on the natural history of untreated cancers which grow, spread and ultimately cause death. Administration of each cycle or dose of treatment kills a substantial proportion of tumour cells (Norton and Simon 1977) and as such is linked to delaying death (Norton 2001). These principles may be applicable to chemotherapeutic agents which target tumour cell kill, and therefore the endpoint of response may be a relevant indicator of anti-tumour activity.

There are inherent issues in the assessment of tumour response, associated with investigator bias, inter-observer reliability and variation in observed response rates over multiple trials (Therasse 2002). These may, to some degree, be alleviated by the incorporation of independent central review of response assessments or the incorporation of a randomised control arm when historical response data are unreliable. The use of classical response criteria for trials of drugs that may not cause tumour shrinkage is likely to be inappropriate and raises questions over the design of phase II trials and the endpoints being used (Twombly 2006). Measures of time to an event such as disease progression or novel endpoints such as biomarkers may be more relevant when evaluating the activity of newer targeted therapies. Nevertheless, because most targeted or biological therapies are selected for clinical development on the basis of pre-clinical data demonstrating at least some degree of tumour regression, tumour response may remain an appropriate outcome measure for novel agents, as acknowledged by two Task Force publications (Booth et al. 2008; Seymour et al. 2010).

2.2.1.2   Continuous

Continuous outcome measures such as tumour volume or biomarker response may be appropriate and relevant outcome measures for consideration in studies of novel agents (Adjei et al. 2009; Karrison et al. 2007; McShane et al. 2009). The use of biomarkers in clinical trials is becoming increasingly common in the development of targeted treatments with novel mechanisms of action. Only when a biomarker has been validated as an outcome measure of activity, that is, when a clear relationship has been established with a more conventional clinically relevant outcome measure, should a biomarker be used as the primary outcome measure of a phase II trial. The difficulties in identifying validated biomarkers have been highlighted (McShane et al. 2009), in addition to the need for technical validation and quality assurance of the relevant assays. As discussed above, biomarkers may be dichotomised to produce a binary outcome; statistical designs can, however, incorporate biomarkers as a continuous outcome, which may often lead to more efficient trial design.

2.2.1.3   Multinomial

Multinomial outcome measures may offer an alternative to binary outcomes when multiple levels of a clinical outcome may be of importance. For targeted or cytostatic therapies, an alternative to binary tumour response (i.e. response vs. no response) that remains objective may be the ordered categories of tumour response such as complete response plus partial response versus stable disease versus progressive disease (Booth et al. 2008; Dhani et al. 2009). Alternatively activity of an experimental therapy may be evidenced by either a sufficiently high response rate or a sufficiently low early progressive disease rate (Sun et al. 2009).

2.2.1.4   Time to event

Time to progression (TTP), time-to-treatment failure (TTF) or PFS may be considered as appropriate outcome measures to assess the activity of treatments in phase II clinical trials (Pazdur 2008).

- TTP may be defined as the time from registration or randomisation into a clinical trial to time of progressive disease;

- TTF may be defined as time from registration/randomisation to treatment discontinuation for any reason, including disease progression, treatment toxicity, patient preference or death;

- PFS may be defined as time from registration/randomisation to objective tumour progression or death.

The use of these endpoints has increased in recent years as a means of assessing the activity of targeted or cytostatic treatments, including cancer vaccines. While TTP and PFS may better capture the activity of such agents, they do present their own challenges. Trials incorporating TTP or PFS as the primary outcome measure may be constrained by a lack of accurate historical time-to-event population data with which to make comparisons. This limitation may be overcome by randomised, comparative designs, but they inherently require larger sample sizes. TTP or PFS may be influenced by assessment bias in terms of frequency of assessment irrespective of randomisation, highlighting the need to carefully consider the schedule of follow-up assessments; increasingly, assessments are recommended at fixed time points rather than in relation to the number of cycles of treatment received to avoid such biases.

Additional time-to-event outcome measures may also be considered including, for example, time to developing an SAE in trials primarily concerned with safety assessment or time to a clinical event such as bone fracture in trials of drugs specifically acting against bone metastases.

2.2.1.5   Ratio of times to progression

One way to overcome the limitations of TTP and PFS as outcome measures with regard to the challenges of unreliable historical data, and to avoid the need for additional patient numbers in a randomised study, may be to use each patient as their own control. The ratio of times to progression or 'growth modulation index' has been proposed for trials in patients who have had at least one previous line of treatment (Mick et al. 2000; Von Hoff 1998).

The growth modulation index (GMI) represents the ratio of the TTP on the current investigational treatment relative to that on the previous line of 'standard' treatment, that is, sequentially measured paired failure times for each patient. Although originally proposed in the 1990s, this outcome measure may be considered exploratory, as it has not been widely used in phase II trials to date and relies on TTP data from the previous line of treatment, the accuracy of which may be uncertain as it will usually have been administered outside a clinical trial when assessments are less structured. A GMI of 1.33 has been proposed as clinically relevant, but this threshold has not been validated (Von Hoff 1998). Time-to-event ratios may, however, be worthy of consideration as a phase II outcome measure where randomisation is not appropriate.

2.2.2   Randomisation

The use of randomisation in phase II trials is widely debated (Buyse 2000; Redman and Crowley 2007; Yothers et al. 2006). Randomisation protects against selection bias, balances treatment groups for prognostic factors and contributes towards ensuring a valid comparison of the treatments under investigation, such that any treatment effect observed can reasonably be attributed to the treatment under investigation and not external confounding factors.

Although randomised phase III clinical trials provide the mainstay of evidence-based clinical research, the use of randomisation within phase II is not so straight-forward. Those opposed to randomisation in phase II trials argue that it can be unacceptably restrictive from a resource perspective, as it inevitably requires at least twice the number of patients (assuming 1:1 randomisation), increasing both the cost and duration of the trial (Yothers et al. 2006). A further criticism is that where the main purpose of randomisation is to balance for potential prognostic factors (of which there may be many), this is unlikely to be achieved in randomised phase II trials that are generally only modest in size (Redman and Crowley 2007). On the other hand, those making the case *for* randomised phase II trials stress the inherent problems of selection bias in uncontrolled trials (Buyse 2000). Therapeutic benefits are generally smaller than potential differences in outcome due to baseline patient and disease characteristics; patient selection bias can, therefore, seriously confound the interpretation of non-randomised phase II trials, and thus the decision to take a treatment forward to phase III. This may not be a problem in a phase IIa trial of a new cytotoxic that is simply screening to establish whether it has a pre-specified, and often low, level of activity; bias is more of a challenge in a phase IIb trial where the key question is whether a new treatment has a sufficiently high level of activity to warrant a large phase III trial.

For an increasing number of phase II studies, especially those of cytostatic or targeted agents, where 'traditional' endpoints such as response rate are not likely to be the most appropriate outcome measures, historical controls are problematic as data for alternative endpoints such as PFS may not be available. Where such data do exist, the population of patients on which the data are available must be considered since patients entering phase II clinical trials will not be representative of the broader patient population treated in routine practice from which historical outcome data may be derived. It is, therefore, important that the patients from whom the historical outcome data are derived are matched as closely as possible to the phase II population in terms of baseline characteristics and disease biomarkers if used for enrichment. If this is not possible, there is a strong argument to include randomisation against a control arm within the phase II trial.

In the context of randomisation, another important point is whether the experimental therapy under investigation is to be delivered as a single agent or in combination. Where an experimental therapy is given in combination with the current standard treatment, it is very difficult to identify any additional activity of the experimental agent over and above that of the standard partner therapy unless a comparative control arm is incorporated into the trial. Even if historical activity data do exist for the standard therapy, patient selection and evolving patterns of patient care may often render the interpretation of such data difficult. This should be considered in detail when making the decision as to whether or not to incorporate a randomised control arm.

Although randomisation is increasingly being incorporated into phase II trial design, it can take various forms. Simply because randomisation between experimental and control treatments is incorporated into a phase II trial does not automatically imply that the two arms are formally statistically compared with sufficient power; the reasons for randomisation should, therefore, be critically evaluated.

The statistical implications of conducting a single-arm or a randomised phase II study have been evaluated in simulation studies. One study compared the results of multi-centre single-arm and randomised phase II trials of the same sample size, where the decision as to whether or not the experimental treatment was deemed successful was based solely on it showing a higher response rate than in the historical control population, or randomised control population, that is, no formally powered statistical comparison was employed (Taylor et al. 2006). Where there was expected to be little variability in response rates between centres, and both the variability and uncertainty in the response rate for the control population were small, single-arm studies were found to be adequate in terms of correct decision-making. However, with increased variability and uncertainty in response rates for either the experimental or control population, randomised studies were more likely to make the correct recommendation regarding proceeding to phase III, and should be considered as a possible option. A further study compared error rates between single-arm and randomised comparative phase II trials, which reflected more realistically the characteristics of a phase II trial (Tang et al. 2010). Although sample sizes for the randomised trials were at least double those of the single-arm trials, the false-positive error rates (type I error) in single-arm trials were two to four times those projected when the characteristics of the study patients differed from those of the historical controls; by contrast, randomised trials remained close to the planned type I error. Statistical power (type II error) remained stable for both designs despite differences in the patient populations.

The impact of misspecification of the control data for either approach should be considered in detail, for example, the impact of specifying a control response rate of, say, 60% when in fact it may be as low as, say, 50%, or as high as 70%. In the single-arm setting, the impact of such misspecification, potentially leading to increased false-negative or false-positive results, is much higher than in the randomised setting since there is no concurrent control arm against which to verify the initial control assumptions made. Thus where there is uncertainty in the control data, the inclusion of a control arm may be considered appropriate.

There is no one-size-fits-all approach to phase II trial design, and the theoretical and practical implications of randomisation must be considered on a trial-by-trial basis. Below we discuss the various randomisation options for phase II trial design and provide examples of when each setting may be appropriate. Randomisation is categorised within the thought process as

i. no randomisation (single-arm phase II trial);

ii. randomisation incorporating a control arm, no formally powered statistical comparison intended;

iii. randomisation incorporating a control arm, formal comparison intended; and

iv. randomisation to multiple experimental treatments.

The use of randomised discontinuation designs is addressed separately in Section 2.2.3.

2.2.2.1   No randomisation

Chapter 3 outlines those designs that incorporate only a single experimental arm. The results of most single-arm phase II trials are interpreted in the context of historical control data. The reliability, or otherwise, of these historical data is one of the main issues driving discussion about randomisation in phase II studies (Rubinstein et al. 2009; Vickers et al. 2007). Single-arm phase II designs have been reported that utilise historical data but incorporate an estimate of potential variability arising from the number of patients or trials from which those historical data have been derived, and are presented in Chapter 3.

A single-arm study may be considered appropriate where

- comparison with a control group is not relevant. For example, a phase IIa trial designed to show proof of concept, where the intention is to obtain an initial estimate of treatment activity to inform the design of a randomised phase IIb trial;

- the historical data are sufficiently robust for the primary outcome measure as to allow a reliable comparison, for example, a study of a single-agent cytotoxic treatment with response rate as the primary outcome measure, conducted in a broad population of patients with a common cancer refractory to standard therapy.

2.2.2.2   Randomisation including a control arm

Randomisation including a control arm can be considered in two ways: randomisation with no formal comparison between experimental and control arms and randomisation *with* a formal comparison between experimental and control arms. Further discussion of each of these is given below. Phase II trial designs incorporating randomisation between a single experimental therapy (or combination therapy) and a control arm are presented in Chapter 4.

With no formal comparison

Those designs that incorporate a control arm with no formal comparison intended as the primary decision-making assessment are highlighted in Chapter 4, as the study is not designed to have sufficient power to detect statistically significant differences between treatment arms. This does not infer that a comparison may not be made of outcomes between the arms; rather, that these comparisons be made with the acknowledgement of reduced statistical power therefore providing additional exploratory comparisons only. This approach may be appropriate if it is sufficient to simply show that the experimental treatment has activity within a certain range. Randomisation provides a level of reassurance that the study population is representative and guards against patient selection bias; this approach is more acceptable when at least some historical data exist to further aid interpretation of the activity of the investigational agent.

In the absence of formal comparison between treatment arms, the sample size may simply be doubled compared to a single-arm study and decision-making at the end of the trial based primarily on the results of the experimental arm, albeit in the context of outcomes in the control arm. Data from the patients randomised to the control arm can be more formally incorporated. For example, response rates in the control arm may be compared to the historical control rates to determine whether they are reflective of the assumptions made when designing the trial (Buyse 2000; Herson and Carter 1986).

It has been suggested that the use of a control arm as a reference arm only should be avoided, particularly in trials of targeted or cytostatic agents, since it may be difficult to interpret the results when unexpected outcomes are observed in the control arm and when the sample size is not sufficient enough to permit direct formally powered comparisons (Rubinstein et al. 2009). For example, if positive results were observed in the experimental arm on the basis of pre-defined criteria, but higher than expected activity was also observed in the control arm, does this call into question the positive trial outcome? On the other hand, if the outcome of the experimental arm is negative and the control arm also has a lower level of activity than expected, should the apparent low activity of the experimental treatment be questioned? These uncertainties may be mitigated by looking at both study arms in relation to appropriate historical data, where available.

With formal comparison

When a phase II trial aims to determine more than whether the investigational agent has activity within a broad range, or there are serious doubts about the accuracy of historical control data, formal comparison between the control and experimental treatment arms is preferred. The trade-off for increased reliability is inevitably a larger sample size.

The level of statistical significance within a comparative, randomised phase II trial should be considered carefully as this will further impact on sample size. It is acceptable to increase the type I error in a phase II trial compared to the typical 5% level used within phase III trials, and error rates of up to 20% have been used. This may enable more realistic sample sizes, and the error associated with incorrectly declaring a non-active treatment worthy of further investigation in phase III (i.e. the type I error) may be deemed more acceptable than that of incorrectly rejecting a treatment that is active. It is, therefore, important to maintain the power associated with the design of the trial.

Another consideration in the use of formally comparative phase II designs is the feasibility of achieving the treatment difference that is being specified. While it may be appropriate to target large treatment effects in some circumstances, this may not be the case in others. The size of the clinically relevant treatment effect should, therefore, be considered carefully to ensure the outcome assumptions are realistic and not simply used as a method of reducing sample size.

It must also be stressed that with the use of formally comparative phase II designs, a statistically significant result at phase II would not usually obviate the need for a subsequent phase III trial. In contrast to the short-term endpoints usually selected in phase II trials, longer term endpoints such as PFS and OS are typically selected in large-scale phase III trials. Additionally, in a relatively small randomised phase II study only a limited number of patients will have received study drug so not all clinically relevant toxicities may be identified and should therefore be studied further. Information gained from the phase II trial may also influence patient selection for the definitive phase III study. Subsequent confirmatory phase III trials are, therefore, usually required even after a statistically positive randomised phase II trial.

2.2.2.3 Randomisation to experimental arms (selection)

Where the aim of a phase II trial is to select which of several candidate investigational treatments to take forward for further evaluation, randomisation may be incorporated to randomise patients between several experimental treatments. Where historical control data are either available or not relevant as discussed above, this will influence the decision as to whether or not a control arm is also incorporated, also as discussed above.

2.2.3 Design category

Phase II statistical designs can be broadly separated into nine statistical design categories:

- one-stage;
- two-stage;
- multi-stage (or group sequential);
- continuous monitoring;
- decision-theoretic;
- three-outcome;
- phase II/III;
- randomised discontinuation; and
- targeted subgroups.

These categories are not mutually exclusive. For example, a one-stage trial may incorporate a three-outcome design, or analysis based on a decision-theoretic approach. Where this is the case, designs have been listed according to their primary design categorisation.

A brief description of these nine categories is provided below, focusing on the practical implementation of each design. Previous reviews have used alternative categories for phase II designs, focusing either on single-arm versus randomised studies (Seymour et al. 2010) or specific designs such as randomised designs, enrichment designs and adaptive Bayesian designs for trials of molecularly targeted agents only (Booth et al. 2008). Mariani and Marubini also previously conducted a review of the statistical methods available for phase II trials, categorising designs according to one sample versus controlled, as well as according to the number of stages of assessments, and focusing on a framework for trial analysis, that is, frequentist, Bayesian or decision theoretic (Mariani and Marubini 1996). The grouping of trial designs within this book adopts a similar design categorisation to Mariani and Marubini (Mariani and Marubini 1996), but the thought process incorporates points for discussion prior to making the specific design decision. Additional categories of design that Mariani and Marubini (Mariani and Marubini 1996) did not consider are also included.

2.2.3.1   One-stage

A one-stage design utilises a fixed sample of patients, recruited until the required sample size is obtained. After the necessary follow-up of patients, analysis and decision-making regarding proof of concept, whether to move to phase III or not, or which treatment(s) to select to take forward to phase III, is made. One-stage designs are relatively straightforward, avoiding complexities relating to recruitment strategies if interim analyses are undertaken. They do not, however, allow for adaptations such as early trial termination due to low levels of activity. Where the safety of a treatment is well known, and data are already available to suggest activity, either for a similar treatment or for the same treatment in an alternative population of patients, a single-stage design may be appropriate since an interim 'check' may be deemed unnecessary.

Where the experimental therapy is highly active, over and above the current standard therapy, fewer patients may be required under a one-stage design than other two- or multi-stage designs that incorporate early termination for lack of activity only.

2.2.3.2   Two-stage

Under a two-stage design patients are recruited to the trial in two stages such that at the end of the first stage an interim analysis is performed and the trial may be stopped for a number of reasons, including lack of activity, early evidence of activity or unacceptable toxicity; otherwise, the trial continues to a second stage. Alternatively, the interim analysis may be used to select which of several experimental treatments to take forward to the second stage. Additional adaptations may be incorporated at the end of the first stage according to the specific trial design, for example, sample size re-estimation.

Stopping rules are developed for each stage of the study to determine whether to stop or continue, based on pre-specified operating characteristics relevant to the specific trial and design. At the end of the study, data from both stages are typically used in deciding how to proceed.

Two-stage designs are beneficial in that the analysis at the end of the first stage may act as a 'check' on the treatment(s) under investigation, potentially exposing fewer patients to an inactive treatment than would be exposed using a one-stage design (i.e. under the null hypothesis of no treatment activity, two-stage designs may be more efficient). There are, however, issues around patient recruitment while data from the first stage of the trial are being analysed. This is a particular issue if the outcome of interest requires a substantial period of follow-up or observation, for example, PFS requiring a specific number of events to be observed. During this time, patients either continue to be recruited, therefore contributing to the second-stage sample size, *without* the results of the first stage being known, or recruitment is suspended. Continuing recruitment avoids the trial losing momentum and may be acceptable where recruitment is slow. If a trial is recruiting rapidly, however, the total required number of patients may be entered to the second stage of the trial before the first-stage analysis is complete, rendering the two-stage design futile.

Careful thought must be given to these points when a two-stage design is being considered. A compromise may be considered, which does not require a break in recruitment but takes into account data from patients recruited during the follow-up and analysis period of the first-stage patients if required (Herndon 1998). If the first-stage analysis suggests stopping due to lack of activity, recruitment may be suspended at this stage and an additional assessment performed incorporating data on all patients recruited during the follow-up and analysis period to determine whether to stop the trial permanently or to resume recruitment (see Chapter 3). Additionally, other two-stage designs can be adapted when the attained sample size is different to the planned sample size, especially if this results in over-recruitment, where the decision-making criteria may be updated in line with the actual number of patients recruited (Chen and Ng 1998; Green and Dahlberg 1992).

Due to the nature of two-stage designs, the total sample size requirement is not fixed, so a maximum sample size and an average sample number (ASN) are generally specified, to account for possible early termination of the trial.

2.2.3.3 Multi-stage

Multi-stage designs, also known as group-sequential designs, are similar to the two-stage designs described above, but with additional analyses throughout the course of the trial. This allows more opportunities to terminate the trial, exposing fewer patients to inactive and/or toxic treatments, or to accelerate the start of the phase III trial through early termination of the phase II trial if sufficient evidence of activity is seen. Additional adaptations may be incorporated at each stage, and again stopping rules are developed for each stage of the study based on pre-specified operating characteristics relevant to the specific trial. As with two-stage designs, multi-stage designs require consideration of whether to continue recruitment whilst interim assessments are underway. Again, due to the nature of multi-stage designs, a maximum sample size and an ASN are generally specified.

Two-stage or multi-stage designs are generally chosen because of their ability to terminate a trial earlier than a fixed sample one-stage design and may be seen to allow a more cautious approach. This is useful when the activity of a treatment is not known and/or toxicity is likely to be considerable. In this case a two-stage or multi-stage design may be appropriate irrespective of the implications of continuing or suspending recruitment. Where such caution is not necessary, a two-stage or multi-stage design may not be appropriate, especially when either suspending or continuing recruitment is problematic; in these cases, a one-stage design may be an alternative.

2.2.3.4 Continuous monitoring

With continuous monitoring designs the outcome of interest is assessed after each individual patient's primary outcome has been observed. The rationale behind this design is generally to allow early termination of the trial in case of lack of activity. This provides, therefore, a more cautious approach to trial design, allowing termination as soon as possible rather than waiting for a pre-defined number of patients to be recruited. Again, pre-defined stopping rules are required and determined via the specific design operating characteristics. Recruitment may continue while the outcomes are observed, but real-time reporting of outcomes is fundamental to this design. This is not possible if the primary outcome requires a prolonged period of observation as with PFS or even best response, both of which may not be available for some months following the start of treatment. In such cases there is little to be gained from continuous monitoring over a multi-stage design, since many additional patients may be recruited before data from the 'last' patient can be analysed. This may be less problematic where, for example, acute treatment toxicity is the key outcome measure, as this can generally be assessed more quickly than activity.

2.2.3.5 Decision-theoretic

Decision-theoretic designs consider costs and gains associated with making incorrect decisions at the end of the phase II trial and incorporate utility functions associated with these costs and gains. Variables such as the total patient 'horizon', that is, the likely number of patients who would be treated with an effective new drug as standard therapy after completion of a successful phase III trial, before the next new, more effective drug becomes available, are required (Sylvester 1988). If that patient population is small, and especially if the likely cost of the new treatment high, there may be a financial imperative that the magnitude of the treatment effect sought in the phase II study be large. Decisions are generally made at the end of the trial after a fixed number of patients have been recruited, as in a one-stage design, although multi-stage designs may also be used. These designs allow decisions to be made based on an all-round assessment of gain, as opposed to concentrating solely on clinical activity (Sylvester and Staquet 1980).

Although the ability to incorporate information regarding costs and gains associated with decisions made throughout a trial is clearly potentially useful, decision-theoretic designs are rarely used in phase II oncology trials. This may reflect the difficulty of identifying accurately the cost and patient horizon information that is often required for their design and difficulty in formulating realistic and interpretable models.

2.2.3.6 Three-outcome

The three-outcome design may be seen as a sub-design of the one-, two- or multi-stage designs (Storer 1992). The main characteristic of this design is that instead of there being two possible outcomes at the end of the phase II trial, that is, reject the null hypothesis or reject the alternative hypothesis, a third outcome is incorporated where the trial is inconclusive on the basis of primary endpoint data. This approach may be used when there is a region of uncertainty between, for example, a response rate above which further investigation in phase III is warranted and a response rate below which it is not. If the primary outcome measure data of such a trial are inconclusive, the decision to move to phase III or not may be based on alternative outcome measures such as safety or cost.

Three-outcome designs may be single arm or randomised. Upper and lower stopping boundaries are developed for each stage of the study to determine whether to stop, continue or declare the trial inconclusive. To calculate these boundaries, in addition to the conventional type I and type II errors (α and β, respectively), two further errors must also be considered. The probability of correctly making the decision to reject the null hypothesis when the alternative is true (π) and the probability of correctly making the decision to reject the alternative hypothesis when the null is true (η), are required. With these four errors specified one can then determine the probability of incorrectly declaring an inconclusive result when in fact the alternative hypothesis is true (δ) and the probability of incorrectly declaring an inconclusive result when in fact the null hypothesis is true (λ). These differing error rates are shown graphically in Figure 2.2, assuming a binary outcome measure of success or failure. Here, n_L and n_U represent the lower and upper stopping boundaries, respectively, for the number of successes observed; N is the sample size; and p_0 and p_1 represent the success rates associated with the null and alternative hypotheses, respectively. Alternatively, the probabilities of concluding in favour of either the null or alternative hypotheses when in fact the true response rate lies within the region of uncertainty may be specified (Storer 1992).

Three-outcome designs generally require fewer patients than a typical two-outcome design using the same design criteria. They may also be seen as better reflecting clinical reality than the typical two-outcome design where the decision

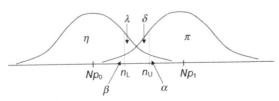

Figure 2.2   Probabilities associated with the three-outcome design.

between accepting and rejecting the null hypothesis may be determined by a single success or failure (i.e. a single stopping boundary).

2.2.3.7 Phase II/III

Phase II/III designs are used when the transition from phase II to III is required to be seamless. Such designs typically allow data generated from the phase II component of the trial to be incorporated in the final phase III analysis. These trials are, therefore, usually randomised, incorporating a control arm. Randomisation may be used to select the 'best' of several treatments in the phase II component to be carried forward into phase III or to decide whether or not to continue an individual experimental treatment (single-agent or combination therapy) into the phase III component.

One of the main benefits of these designs is that they reduce the total time required for the study to progress through phases II and III compared to running separate trials. Since data from the phase II component may also be incorporated in the phase III analysis, patient resources are also reduced; this is a major benefit in rarer cancers or disease sub-types where the patient population is small. Where a limited number of patients are available for trial recruitment, the optimal use of patient data is even more crucial than usual.

Alternatively, where separate phase II and phase III trials are to be carried out, a phase II trial allowing early termination for evidence of activity may be considered appropriate, bringing forward the phase III trial and saving patient resource. Where patient numbers are limited, various trial design scenarios should be investigated to identify the design which is most efficient in terms of patient numbers whilst providing sufficiently robust results.

As with multi-stage designs, the issue of whether to continue or suspend recruitment during the analysis of the phase II component arises. The trial risks losing momentum if recruitment is suspended, but rapid recruitment during this period may result in a substantial number of patients being entered into the phase III element, rendering the phase II/III design futile in its attempts to reduce the number of patients exposed prior to embarking on phase III. For these trials to be carried out successfully, the funding body, be it academic or industry, must commit to the full phase II/III package in the knowledge that the trial may terminate after the phase II component. Often many more centres will participate in the phase III component than in the phase II. Since the trial may terminate for lack of activity after the phase II component, the early preparation of centre set-up to enable a smooth transition to phase III must be weighed against this possibility of early termination.

Specific phase II/III designs are outlined in Chapters 3–7. An alternative approach to designing a phase II/III trial is to use conventional stand-alone phase II designs to make decisions as to whether to continue to phase III or not and incorporate these into phase III seamlessly (Storer 1990). Typically in this case, the primary outcome measure under investigation during phase II is different to the primary outcome measure under investigation during the phase III component, to avoid the need to adjust the type I error rate in the phase III component. Otherwise, when the same outcome measure is used in both phases II and III, with a formal comparison between control and experimental treatments at the end of phase II, this essentially becomes a phase III trial with at least one interim analysis. This approach, using the same endpoints, is not generally recommended since the phase III endpoint will usually be a long-term outcome such as OS. A long follow-up period would, therefore, be required for that endpoint to be assessed in the interim/phase II analysis. Multi-stage approaches may, however, be based on the phase II outcome measure with subsequent interim analyses within the phase III component based on the phase III endpoints.

Phase II/III designs are inevitably associated with patient and resource efficiencies, accelerating the transition between the two trial phases, and usually allowing patients recruited to phase II to be incorporated in the phase III analysis. However, by performing separate phase II and phase III trials the results of the phase II trial, and lessons learned during its set-up and conduct, may be incorporated into the design of the phase III trial. Changes to eligibility criteria or follow-up schedules, for example, may be required for the phase III trial. Here separate phase II and III trials enable these alterations to be made. Such an approach to the planning of current and future trials may be beneficial where experience with an experimental treatment is minimal, or data for the control population of the disease area in question are minimal, enabling additional learning between stages of the development pathway.

2.2.3.8   Randomised discontinuation

Randomised discontinuation, or enrichment, trial designs (Kopec et al. 1993; Rosner et al. 2002; Stadler 2007) involve all study patients initially being treated with the experimental treatment for a pre-defined period of time, and then assessed for response to treatment. Typically, those with progressive disease come off study whilst patients who are responding continue to receive the experimental agent; those with stable disease are randomised to either continue the experimental treatment or discontinue it and either remain off treatment or receive standard treatment depending on the question being asked in the trial.

Such an approach may be appropriate when the specific population of patients in which the experimental treatment is expected to be effective is unknown. For example, when evaluating a targeted agent where the level of expression of the relevant target required for potential activity is not known, a randomised discontinuation design may allow *de facto* enrichment of the patient population. Against this, only a limited proportion of the population recruited to the trial actually contributes to the randomised part of the study. An overview of the randomised discontinuation design is presented by Stadler, providing an example of where the design has been used successfully, as well as providing a summary of the advantages and disadvantages of the design (Stadler 2007).

The role of the randomised discontinuation design has been reviewed in detail (Booth et al. 2008; Capra 2004; Freidlin and Simon 2005; Kopec et al. 1993; Rosner et al. 2002; Rubinstein et al. 2009). The Methodology for the Development of Innovative Cancer Therapies (MDICT) Task Force (Booth et al. 2008) considered the design as being exploratory in nature due to lack of clarity on its role in oncology. One study comparing the randomised discontinuation design with a comparative randomised design showed that the randomised discontinuation design may be underpowered in comparison to the traditional design due to the number of patients who start the investigational treatment who are not then randomised (Capra 2004). An accurate estimate of the proportion of patients likely to enter randomisation is, therefore, essential in planning the study sample size. By contrast, a second study concluded that, although the randomised discontinuation design may be less efficient than the classical randomised design in many settings, it can be useful in the early development of targeted agents where a reliable assay to select patients expressing the target is not available (Freidlin and Simon 2005). The randomised discontinuation design may be especially appropriate when treatment benefit is restricted to a select group of patients who are not identifiable at the start of the trial.

2.2.3.9   Targeted subgroups

In the era of targeted therapies it may be appropriate to investigate the activity of a treatment in a specific subgroup of patients in whom the intervention is anticipated to be effective. Alternatively, where the specific subgroup of patients is not determined, or there is uncertainty about whether a biomarker accurately identifies a 'sensitive' patient population, it may be appropriate to assess activity simultaneously in several subgroups of patients according to biomarker characterisation. Population enrichment for a specific biomarker in phase II trials was discussed in Section 2.1.1.4, highlighting the risks associated with incorrect characterisation and the possibilities of false-negative results, as well as issues surrounding the use of historical data.

Designs that incorporate subgroup stratification may be used to enable the inclusion of separate cohorts of patients defined by the biomarker in question, or populations defined by other disease sub-types or patient characteristics, ensuring that adequate numbers are recruited into each cohort. Approaches incorporating stratification range from separate phase II trials within each stratification level, to hierarchical Bayesian designs (Thall et al. 2003) and tandem two-stage methods where the experimental treatment is first tested in an unselected patient population, and if there is insufficient activity in this overall group, the trial continues in a select population (e.g. marker-positive patients) only (Pusztai et al. 2007). Trials may also be partially enriched to include a larger proportion of, for example, biomarker-positive patients, providing additional power to detect treatment effects in this targeted subgroup of patients.

These designs are discussed in Chapter 7; however, as noted in Chapter 1, a number of recent papers have been published on biomarker stratification (An et al. 2012; Buyse et al. 2011; Freidlin et al. 2012; Freidlin and Korn 2013; Jenkins et al. 2011; Lai et al. 2012; Mandrekar et al. 2013; Roberts and Ramakrishnan 2011; Tournoux-Facon et al. 2011), therefore we encourage consideration of additional literature outlining alternative designs available.

2.3   Stage 3 – Practicalities

2.3.1   Practical considerations

At this stage of the design process, when faced with a number of statistical designs from which to choose, deciding which particular design is most appropriate to your particular setting can be difficult. Although all the designs considered are deemed easy to implement, this section focuses on key practical aspects.

2.3.1.1 Programming requirements

For each statistical design described in Chapters 3–7, the programming require-ments have been considered. It is important that the statistical methodology can be implemented easily and efficiently, allowing the statistician to consider various trial scenarios during the design process. Only those designs that detail availability of programs, or for which sufficient information is provided to allow the design to be implemented, have been incorporated in this book. Nevertheless, some designs may still be easier to implement than others depending on the resources available.

2.3.1.2 Availability/robustness of prior data

It is essential to consider the design parameters that must be defined in order to implement each design and the variability associated with each of these parameters. There may be, for example, a paucity of data on the primary outcome measure for patients receiving the current standard treatment in the particular trial setting, so what is the impact of those historical data being unreliable? For example, if the response rate with standard therapy is estimated to be 20%, a phase II study may aim for a response rate of 30% with the experimental arm. If a randomised phase II trial is powered on such a basis but the patients in the control arm have better outcomes than expected, the study may be underpowered. On the other hand, if a single-arm study is undertaken and the historical response rate is overestimated an active treatment may be inappropriately discarded. The implication of misspecification of study parameters may be investigated by simulation or may already be addressed within the specific design publication. If a trial design is not robust with regard to misspecification, it may be more appropriate to consider a design that allows either an estimate of the variance of the parameter to be incorporated into the design or to select a different outcome measure that is robust in the face of misspecification. Additionally there may be a specific design parameter for which no reliable data are available, for example, an estimate of the correlation between a change in a biomarker and a clinically relevant outcome measure. Here it may be possible either to consider a design that does not require the parameter in question or to simulate the performance of the design under differing parameter assumptions.

2.3.1.3 Early termination

Typically in phase II trials, early termination of a trial is incorporated to ensure the safety and appropriate treatment of patients, usually in the context of lack of activity or unacceptable toxicity. Early termination when evidence of activity has been demonstrated may not be deemed necessary given the desire to obtain as much information on the treatment as possible to provide a more robust estimate of the treatment's activity to inform the design of subsequent trials. On the other hand, this may delay opening of subsequent phase III trials and there are designs that do incorporate early termination for activity.

2.3.1.4 Operating characteristics

In phase II trials, a larger type I error than typically used in phase III trials (e.g. 5% two sided) is generally accepted due to the nature of phase II trials. Type I errors of up to 20% have been used where the consequences of incorrectly rejecting an active treatment are deemed less acceptable than those of inappropriately continuing to develop a treatment that will ultimately not be active. In such circumstances, subsequent larger phase III studies would be expected to identify the treatment as inactive, whereas if a treatment is rejected the situation may well not be remedied as a phase III trial is unlikely. The selection of an appropriate type I error rate is, therefore, crucial to the reliability of the trial results and the efficient development of new treatments. While larger type I error rates allow smaller sample sizes, investigators need to consider carefully whether it is appropriate to conduct a small phase II study with a high risk of a false-positive result, and 'negative' subsequent phase III trial; the alternative is a larger phase II study with a lesser chance of development of an ultimately 'negative' phase III trial.

Since the primary aim of many phase II trials is to determine whether a treatment has a pre-specified level of activity, the power of phase II studies should generally remain high; in practice, this means a power of at least 80%.

2.4 Summary

This chapter provides guidance on decision-making when identifying a trial design for a phase II trial (Figure 2.1). Clinical researchers and statisticians should consider carefully each of the three stages of the thought process; additional resources should be consulted where necessary, and discussion maintained between the clinician and statistician. The guidance we offer is not intended to be exhaustive or proscriptive. Further reading and discussion around specific areas relevant to each specific phase II design element should always be encouraged.

Examples of using the thought process in practice are presented in Chapters 8–12 for various trial design scenarios. These are intended as practical examples of how the thought process may be implemented.

3

Designs for single experimental therapies with a single arm

Sarah Brown

3.1 One-stage designs

3.1.1 Binary outcome measure

Fleming (1982)

- One-stage, binary outcome

- Standard software available

Fleming proposes a one-stage, two-stage and multi-stage design requiring specification of response rates under the null and alternative hypotheses and type I and II error rates. Decision criteria are based around rejecting the null hypothesis that the response rate of the experimental treatment is not less than some pre-specified response rate, typically defined as the expected response rate of the current historical control treatment. Sample size is based on normal approximation to the binomial distribution. This is a widely used design and programs are readily available (e.g. Machin et al. 2008).

Fazzari et al. (2000)

- One-stage, binary outcome

- Requires programming

A Practical Guide to Designing Phase II Trials in Oncology, First Edition.
Sarah R. Brown, Walter M. Gregory, Chris Twelves and Julia Brown.
© 2014 John Wiley & Sons, Ltd. Published 2014 by John Wiley & Sons, Ltd.

Fazzari and colleagues propose modifications to previously published phase II designs. The modifications include: incorporating a patient population that is more representative of the intended phase III trial population, by reducing the eligibility restrictions and increasing the number of centres; increasing the sample size to allow more accurate estimates of the treatment activity; using an outcome measure that is more representative of that to be used in phase III, recommending a k-year progression-free survival (PFS) or overall survival (binary) outcome measure for advanced-stage disease populations; taking the upper limit of the 75% confidence interval of the activity of previous treatments as the minimum activity required to be observed to warrant moving to phase III. The methodology for the design of the study is based on rejecting the minimum activity required from an $x\%$ confidence interval around the estimate of treatment activity with, say, 80% probability. Sample size is generated using Monte Carlo simulation which will require programming.

A'Hern (2001)

- One-stage, binary outcome

- Standard software available

A'Hern presents an adaptation of Fleming's design (Fleming 1982). Calculation of sample sizes and cut-offs is based on exact binomial distributions as opposed to normal approximation. Trials based on exact distributions are typically larger than those using the normal approximation; however, they avoid the possibility that confidence intervals around the estimate of activity at the end of the trial will incorrectly contain the lower rejection proportion due to approximation to the normal distribution. As for Fleming, this design is widely used and programs are readily available for its implementation. The choice between Fleming and A'Hern should be based on the sample sizes and the requirement for exact testing.

Chang et al. (2004)

- One-stage, binary outcome

- Pascal programs noted as being available from authors

Chang and colleagues propose a design whereby the sample size, and thus the test statistic, is calculated using exact unconditional methods. This design may be used when the historical control data are based on only a few patients (say up to 120). The number of patients on which the historical data are based is required to be known as analyses take into account the pooled variance of the historical control and experimental data. Tables and software are available to calculate sample sizes.

Mayo and Gajewski (2004)

- One-stage, binary outcome

- Requires programming

Mayo and Gajewski propose sample size calculations for a single-arm single-stage trial with binary outcome, using Bayesian informative priors (pessimistic/optimistic). This is an extension of the two-stage designs proposed by Tan and Machin (2002). Prior information regarding expected response rate and level of uncertainty in this value is required to determine sample sizes using either the mode, median or mean approach. Programming is required for the median and mean approaches, possible in Matlab. Sample sizes will vary depending on the approach used.

Gajewski and Mayo (2006)

- One-stage, binary outcome

- Requires programming

Gajewski and Mayo describe Bayesian sample size calculations where conflicting opinions on prior information can be incorporated. Information required to design the trial includes prior distributions, cut-off for the posterior probability that the true response rate is greater than some pre-specified value and an error term relating to a small increase in the target response rate. Sample size calculation is iterative; therefore some computation is required to identify the design characteristics, for which no software is detailed but for which formulae are given to enable implementation. This design differs from the earlier design proposed by Mayo and Gajewski (2004) as it allows incorporation of pessimistic *and* optimistic priors, as opposed to one informative prior.

Vickers (2009)

- One-stage, binary outcome

- Stata programs given in appendix to manuscript

Vickers proposes a design using historical control data to generate a statistical prediction model for phase II trial. The observed trial data for the experimental arm are then compared to the predicted results to give an indication of whether patients treated with the experimental agents are doing better than expected, based on the prediction model. The authors note that the methodology hinges on quality historical control data relevant to the patient population under study. Step-by-step methodology is presented which incorporates bootstrapping on both the historical data set and the observed data set and a comparison of the predicted and actual outcomes. Example Stata code is given in the appendix to the manuscript to allow implementation of the statistical analysis, as well as assessment of power.

3.1.2 Continuous outcome measure

No references identified.

3.1.3   Multinomial outcome measure

Zee et al. (1999)

- One-stage, multinomial outcome

- Requires programming

Zee and colleagues propose single-stage and multi-stage single-arm designs considering a multinomial outcome, in the context of incorporating progressive disease as well as response into the primary outcome measure. Analysis is based on the number of responses and progressions observed, compared with predetermined stopping criteria. A computer program written in SAS identifies the operating characteristics of the designs. This is not noted as being available in the paper; however, detail is given to allow implementation.

Lu et al. (2005)

- One-stage, multinomial outcome

- Programs may be available from authors

Lu and colleagues propose a design (one-stage or two-stage) to look at both complete response (CR) and total response (or other such outcome measures whereby observing one outcome implies the other outcome is also observed). The design recommends a treatment for further investigation if either of the alternative hypotheses is met (i.e. for CR or for total response) and rejects the treatment if neither is met. The designs follow the general approach of Fleming's single-stage (Fleming 1982) or Simon's two-stage (Simon 1989) approach whereby the number of CRs and total responses are compared to identified stopping boundaries. Tables are provided for some combinations of null and alternative hypotheses; however, formulae are given and at the time of manuscript publication programs were in development. The design differs from others in this section in that one outcome measure is a sub-outcome measure of the other, whereas other designs consider discrete outcome measures such as partial response (PR) versus CR.

Chang et al. (2007)

- One-stage, multinomial outcome

- Programs noted as being available from authors

Chang and colleagues propose a single-stage and a two-stage design for window studies which aim to assess the potential activity of a new treatment in newly diagnosed patients. Treatment is given to patients for a short period of time before standard chemotherapy, and each patient is assessed for response or early progression (both binary outcome measures). The alternative hypothesis is based on both the response rate being above a pre-specified rate *and* the early progressive disease rate being below a pre-specified rate. The outcomes follow a multinomial distribution. A SAS program is noted as being available from the authors to identify designs.

Stallard and Cockey (2008)

- One-stage, multinomial outcome
- Programs noted as being available from author

Stallard and Cockey propose single-arm, one- and two-stage designs for ordered categorical data, where the rejection region for the null hypothesis is defined based on the likelihood ratio test. The null region over which the type I error is controlled considers a weighting of the proportion of patients in each response category, in a similar manner to that of Lin and Chen (2000). The focus of the paper is on response with three levels; however, the design may be extended to more than three levels. Programs are noted as being available from the first author to allow identification of designs.

3.1.4   Time-to-event outcome measure

No references identified.

3.1.5   Ratio of times to progression

Mick et al. (2000)

- One-stage, ratio of times to progression
- Requires programming

Mick and colleagues propose a design based on the growth modulation index (ratio of time to progression of experimental treatment relative to that on the patients' previous course of anti-cancer treatment). The outcome measure is novel and the authors justify its use for trials of cytostatic treatments where outcome measures such as tumour response may not be appropriate. Various values of the growth modulation index for null and alternative hypotheses should be considered to explore design parameters, as appropriate for the setting of the study. Each patient acts as their own control. Information is required for each patient on their time to progression on previous treatment, and an estimate of the correlation between the two times is needed. The design is identified via simulation, which allows investigation of the effect of the correlation estimate on the overall design. Although software is not detailed as being available, this has been implemented in Splus, and detail is provided to allow design implementation.

3.2   Two-stage designs

3.2.1   Binary outcome measure

Gehan (1961)

- Two-stage, binary outcome

- Standard software available

- Early termination for lack of activity

Gehan proposes one of the earliest designs to assess experimental treatments in phase II trials. The methodology is based on the double sampling method and considers a phase II trial composed of a 'preliminary' stage and a 'follow-up' stage. The preliminary stage assesses whether the treatment under investigation is likely to be worth further investigation, using a confidence interval approach to exclude treatments with response rates below those of interest from further investigation. The follow-up stage assesses the activity of the treatment with pre-specified precision. The number of patients to be included in the follow-up stage is determined according to the number of responses observed during the first stage. The proposed design is intended to completely reject inactive treatments quickly, such that if the response rate of interest is excluded from the confidence interval at the end of the first stage, the trial is terminated early. Otherwise the trial continues. In the second stage the activity of the treatment is estimated with given precision, rather than providing decision criteria for continuing to a further trial. On this basis, this design may be seen as an estimation procedure for initial proof of concept trials rather than trials to determine whether or not to proceed to phase III.

Fleming (1982)

- Two-stage, binary outcome

- Standard software available for overall sample size

- Early termination for activity or lack of activity

Fleming proposes a one-stage, two-stage and multi-stage design. The multi-stage design addresses multiple testing considerations to allow early termination in case of extreme results, employing the standard single-stage test procedure at the last test. Tables are presented for specific design scenarios using the exact underlying binomial probabilities rather than the normal approximation to these probabilities. Programs are readily available to calculate the overall sample size for a one-stage design (e.g. Machin et al. 2008), with sample sizes at each stage chosen to be approximately equal. Termination at the end of each stage is permitted for activity or lack of activity.

Simon (1987)

- Two-stage, binary outcome

- Requires programming

- Early termination for lack of activity

Simon introduces a two-stage design that is single arm with a binary outcome whereby the sample size is minimised under a pre-specified expected response rate, not necessarily the null or alternative response rate. Where this expected response rate corresponds with the null hypothesis response rate, this design is equivalent to the optimal design proposed in the subsequent paper summarised below (Simon 1989). The current design is optimised by keeping the size of the first stage small, making the probability of rejecting an inactive drug high, and not allowing too high a sample size in the second stage. Early termination is permitted at the end of stage 1 only for lack of activity. A table is provided with limited design scenarios; however, the designs detailed below (Simon's optimal and minimax) are more widely used and may be considered ahead of this earlier design.

Simon (1989)

- Two-stage, binary outcome

- Standard software available

- Early termination for lack of activity

Simon proposes a single-arm two-stage design based on minimising the expected number of patients under the null hypothesis (optimal), as well as an additional design that minimises the maximum sample size (minimax). This is a well-known and widely used two-stage design, based on null and alternative response rates, power and significance level, and the observed number of responses at the end of each stage is used to assess stopping rules. The outcome of interest is binary and the trial may only be terminated at the end of the first stage for lack of activity. Extensive tables are provided for different design scenarios and software is readily available (e.g. Machin et al. 2008).

Green and Dahlberg (1992)

- Two-stage, binary outcome

- Requires programming

- Early termination for lack of activity

The design described by Green and Dahlberg permits early termination for lack of activity at the end of stage 1 when the alternative hypothesis is rejected at the 0.02 significance level. At the end of the second stage a significance level of 0.055 is used to reject the null hypothesis and declare sufficient activity for further investigation. Some detail is given regarding stopping boundary and sample size calculation, although this would need to be programmed and solved iteratively to find the most suitable design. This paper also discusses adaptations to the designs of Gehan (1961), Fleming (1982), and Simon (1989), in the cases where the final attained trial sample size differs from the original planned design.

Heitjan (1997)

- Two-stage, binary outcome
- Programs noted as being available from the author
- Early termination for activity or lack of activity

Heitjan proposes a design whereby decision-making is based on the ability to persuade someone with extreme prior beliefs that the treatment under investigation is either active or not. This requires specification of extreme priors. For a sceptic, the probability that the experimental treatment is better than the standard treatment must be at least some pre-specified value (e.g. 70%) for the treatment to be declared active (known as the 'persuade the pessimist probability' PPP), and for an enthusiast, the probability that the experimental treatment is worse than the standard treatment must be at least some pre-specified value (e.g. 70%) for the treatment to be declared inactive (known as the 'persuade the optimist probability' POP). Timing of interim analyses can either be based on numbers of patients or time during the trial. Sample size is justified by assessing the operating characteristics and calculating PPPs and POPs of the design under various scenarios. Programs are noted as being available upon request from the author. Early termination is permitted for activity or lack of activity.

Herndon (1998)

- Two-stage, binary outcome
- Requires programming
- Early termination for lack of activity

Herndon proposes a hybrid two-stage design that allows continuation of recruitment while the results of the first stage are being analysed. If the results of the first stage indicate the treatment is inactive, accrual is suspended and data are re-analysed including data from all patients recruited to that time point. Otherwise, the design continues to target recruitment for the second stage. The sample sizes for the first and second stages are chosen for practicality rather than via Simon's optimal method, with overall sample size calculated to maintain pre-specified type I and II errors for study-specific null and alternative hypotheses. Critical values for suspending recruitment, reinitiating or terminating recruitment and for declaring the treatment worthy of further investigation at the end of stage 2 are calculated. To identify the critical values a numerical search is required, for which formulae are provided. If the stage

I results indicate re-analysis using all patients to that time point, analysis follows similar methodology to that proposed by Green and Dahlberg (1992), detailed above, as does the analysis of stage II.

Chen and Ng (1998)

- Two-stage, binary outcome
- Programs noted as being available from authors
- Early termination for lack of activity

Chen and Ng propose a flexible design that operates in the same manner as Simon's two-stage design (Simon 1989), but here the number of patients at the first and second stages can vary by up to eight patients to allow a period of grace in halting recruitment (in a similar manner to that described by Green and Dahlberg 1992, detailed above). A FORTRAN program is noted as being available from the authors to enable implementation, and tables are given for some scenarios.

Chang et al. (1999)

- Two-stage, binary outcome
- Requires programming
- Early termination for activity or lack of activity

Chang and colleagues outline a design for continuous or binary outcomes that takes into account the number of patients on whom historical control data are based. This reflects the fact that the variances of the historical control data and the experimental data will differ. The trial may be terminated at the end of the first stage for either activity or lack of activity. Algorithms are used to determine critical values for stopping, and sample size is calculated by multiplying the single-stage sample size (formulae provided) by between 1.02 and 1.05.

Hanfelt et al. (1999)

- Two-stage, binary outcome
- Programs noted as being available from authors
- Early termination for lack of activity

Hanfelt and colleagues propose a modification to Simon's two-stage design (Simon 1989) that minimises the median number of patients required under the null hypothesis, as opposed to the expected number of patients. A program is noted as being available from the authors that performs the design search. The design differs very little to that of Simon, other than when the response rate of the treatment is much less than the null hypothesis rate. Termination at the end of the first stage is for lack of activity only.

Shuster (2002)

- Two-stage, binary outcome

- Requires programming

- Early termination for activity or lack of activity

The minimax design proposed by Shuster follows the same format as, for example, Simon's design (Simon 1989), although it allows early termination for activity at the end of the first stage, as well as for lack of activity. Sample sizes and cut-offs are calculated based on exact type I and II errors, and the smallest expected maximum sample size is calculated. The author shows that the proposed design generates the smallest sample sizes under the null, alternative and maximum scenarios, compared to Chang et al. (1987) and Fleming (1982). The author advises use of the proposed minimax design when early termination for activity is beneficial (giving as an example the setting of paediatric cancer). A table of specific design scenarios is presented; otherwise the design will require programming.

Tan and Machin (2002)

- Two-stage, binary outcome

- Standard software available

- Early termination for lack of activity

Tan and Machin propose two Bayesian designs: the single threshold design (STD) and the dual threshold design (DTD). The designs are intended to be user-friendly and easily interpreted by those familiar with frequentist phase II designs. They provide an alternative approach to the design, analysis and interpretation of phase II trial data, allowing incorporation of relevant prior information and summarising results in terms of the probability that a response proportion falls within a pre-specified region of interest. The following design parameters are required: target response rate for a new treatment; prior distribution for the experimental treatment being tested; the minimum probability of the true response rate being at least the target response rate at the end of stage 1 (for the STD, $\lambda1$) and at the end of the study ($\lambda2$). For the DTD, the lower response rate of no further interest is also required, and here $\lambda1$ represents the probability that the true response rate is lower than the rate of no further interest at the end of stage 1.

The STD focuses on ensuring, at the end of the first stage, that the final response rate of the drug has a reasonable probability of passing the target response rate at the end of the trial. The DTD, however, focuses on ensuring, at the end of the first stage, that the final response rate at the end of the trial is not below the response rate of no further interest. Tables are given for a number of design scenarios and the designs are compared with the frequentist approach of Simon (1989). Programs have been developed and are available in Machin et al. (2008).

Case and Morgan (2003)

- Two-stage, binary outcome

- Standard software available and programs noted as being available from authors

- Early termination for lack of activity

Case and Morgan outline a design with survival outcomes which are dichotomised to give survival probabilities at pre-specified time points of interest, incorporating all available information. The design is aimed to avoid the drawbacks of extended follow-up periods and breaks in recruitment during follow-up between stages. The design does not require a halt in recruitment between stages as Nelson–Aalen estimates of survival are used to incorporate all survival information up to the time point of interest, at the time of interim analysis. Early termination is permitted only for lack of activity. FORTRAN programs are noted as being available upon request from the authors, to identify the optimal design, and the proposed design is also available in Machin et al. (2008).

Jung et al. (2004)

- Two-stage, binary outcome

- Programs noted as being available from authors

- Early termination for activity or lack of activity

Jung and colleagues propose a searching algorithm to identify admissible two-stage designs based on Bayesian decision theory, incorporating a loss function which is a weighted function of the expected number of patients and the maximum number of patients required. A computer program, developed in Java and noted as being available upon request from the authors, searches admissible designs (comparing the expected loss to the Bayes risk) using information provided on the response rates under null and alternative hypotheses, type I and II errors and maximum number of patients available. Stopping rules are generated based on a minimum number of responses required to be observed.

Lin and Shih (2004)

- Two-stage, binary outcome

- Programs noted as being available from authors

- Early termination for lack of activity

Lin and Shih propose an adaptive design which allows sample size to be adjusted at the end of the first stage, to account for uncertainty in the response rate under the alternative hypothesis. Two potential response rates are pre-specified at the design stage, and the adjustment made based on these. Tables are provided and software is noted as being available from the authors to compute sample size and cut-offs that are not displayed.

Wang et al. (2005)

- Two-stage, binary outcome
- Requires programming
- Early termination for lack of activity

Wang and colleagues propose a Bayesian version of Simon's two-stage design (Simon 1989), controlling frequentist type I and II error rates, as well as Bayesian error rates measured using posterior distributions. The design therefore allows incorporation of commonly controlled error rates familiar with frequentists, as well as enabling calculation of posterior probabilities regarding treatment activity. Stopping at the end of stage I is permitted for lack of activity only. Sample sizes and stopping boundaries for each stage are provided in tables for specific design scenarios, and the design is compared with that of Simon (1989) and the STD and DTDs of Tan and Machin (2002). The design requires programming to enable implementation.

Banerjee and Tsiatis (2006)

- Two-stage, binary outcome
- Programs noted as being available from authors
- Early termination for activity or lack of activity

Banerjee and Tsiatis propose an adaptive design that is similar to Simon's optimal design (Simon 1989); however, the sample size and decision criteria of the second stage depend on the outcome of the first stage, and the trial may terminate at the end of the first stage for either activity or lack of activity. The sample size and decision criteria of the second stage are computed using Bayesian decision theory, minimising the average sample size under the null hypothesis. The design offers a small sample size reduction over Simon's optimal design (3–5%); however, the authors note potential difficulties in planning a trial where the total sample size is unknown at the outset. Tables are given for various design scenarios, and software is noted as being available on request.

Ye and Shyr (2007)

- Two-stage, binary outcome
- Programs available on website
- Early termination for lack of activity

The design proposed by Ye and Shyr follows that of Simon (1989) but is designed to balance the number of patients investigated in each of the stages. Attention is focused on a binary response outcome measure although the design may be extended to multiple correlated outcome measures (where more than one outcome can occur for one patient). Tables are provided with various design scenarios and software is available at www.vicc.org/biostatistics/ts/freqapp.php (last accessed August 2013). The authors note that when there are few patients available, Simon's minimax design would be preferable. If the optimal and minimax designs have dramatically imbalanced sample sizes between the two stages then the proposed design may be preferable; otherwise Simon's optimal design can be used as this minimises the sample size under the null hypothesis. Termination at the end of the first stage is for lack of activity only.

Litwin et al. (2007)

- Two-stage, binary outcome
- Programs noted as being available from authors
- Early termination for activity or lack of activity

Litwin and colleagues describe a design based on the outcome measure of PFS at two set time points. In the second stage of the design the success rate of a binary outcome measure at a set time point $t2$ is considered, which is dependent upon the success rate of a, possibly different, binary outcome measure at an earlier set time point $t1$ (assessed at the end of stage 1), for example, the progression-free rate at time $t2$, dependent upon the progression-free rate at time $t1$. The design incorporates the possibility of stopping for either activity or lack of activity at the end of the first stage and proceeds as follows:

1. $n1$ patients are recruited to the study and followed to time $t1$ for PFS.

2. If there are too few patients who are progression-free at time $t1$ then the trial is stopped early for lack of activity.

3. If there are sufficient patients who are progression-free at time $t1$ then accrual continues to the second stage until a total of $n2$ patients are recruited. Patients in the initial cohort who are progression-free at $t1$ continue on in the study.

4. At the end of the second stage ($t2$) all $n2 - n1$ patients from the second stage and all those patients progression-free at $t1$ are evaluated at time $t2$.

Programs are noted as being available upon request from the authors.

Wu and Shih (2008)

- Two-stage, binary outcome
- Requires programming for adaptations
- Early termination for lack of activity

Wu and Shih propose approaches to handling data that deviate from the pre-specified Simon's two-stage design (Simon 1989). The following scenarios are considered:

- Simon's design 'interrupted', such that there is additional evaluation at the following times:

  a. before completion of the first stage;

  b. after the first stage but before completion of the second stage;

  c. before completion of the first stage and again before completion of the second stage.

- Simon's design 'abandoned', that is, the first unscheduled assessment leads to abandoning the original design and an adapted assessment schedule is developed.

Adaptations to stopping rules are presented as well as detail regarding adjusting the p-value associated with decision-making under the deviated scenario. Adaptations are based on the conditional probability of passing the first stage and the conditional power of rejecting the null hypothesis assuming the study continues to its final stage. No software is detailed; however, sufficient detail is given to allow the design to be programmed for implementation.

Koyama and Chen (2008)

- Two-stage, binary outcome

- Programs available on website

- Early termination for lack of activity

Koyama and Chen detail an adaptation to Simon's two-stage design (Simon 1989) to allow proper inference when the actual sample size at stage 2 deviates from the planned sample size. The methodology allows computation of updated critical values for the second stage, based on the number of responses observed in the first stage, and adapted p-values, point estimates and confidence intervals, incorporating conditional power. Software is available at http://biostat.mc.vanderbilt.edu/wiki/Main/TwoStageInference (last accessed August 2013).

Chi and Chen (2008)

- Two-stage, binary outcome

- Standard programs available as per Simon's two-stage design (Simon 1989)

- Early termination for activity or lack of activity

Chi and Chen propose a curtailed sampling adaptation to Simon's two-stage design (Simon 1989). The design allows earlier termination of the trial in the event that the treatment is either very active or very inactive. Detail of the proposed adaptations is presented and is easily implemented, using standard software to identify a design via Simon's methodology (Simon 1989). The design can offer substantial savings in sample sizes when compared to continuing recruitment to the predetermined number of patients under Simon's design.

Sambucini (2008)

- Two-stage, binary outcome
- Programs noted as being available
- Early termination for lack of activity

Sambucini proposes a Bayesian design which represents a predictive version of the STD proposed by Tan and Machin (2002), taking into account the uncertainty about the data that have not yet been observed, to identify optimal two-stage sample sizes and cut-off values. A 'design' prior and an 'analysis' prior are required to be specified to compute prior predictive distributions and posterior probabilities of treatment activity, respectively. A program written in R is available to determine optimal two-stage designs.

3.2.2   Continuous outcome measure

Chang et al. (1999)

- Two-stage, continuous outcome
- Requires programming
- Early termination for activity or lack of activity

Chang and colleagues outline a design for continuous or binary outcomes that takes into account the number of patients on whom historical control data are based. This reflects the fact that the variances of the historical control data and the experimental data will differ. The trial may be terminated at the end of the first stage for either activity or lack of activity. Algorithms are used to determine critical values for stopping, and sample size is calculated by multiplying the single-stage sample size (formulae provided) by between 1.02 and 1.05.

3.2.3   Multinomial outcome measure

Zee et al. (1999)

- Two-stage, multinomial outcome
- Requires programming
- Early termination for activity or lack of activity

Zee and colleagues propose single-stage and multi-stage single-arm designs considering a multinomial outcome, in the context of incorporating progressive disease as well as response into the primary outcome measure. Analysis is based on the number of responses and progressions observed, compared with predetermined stopping criteria. A computer program written in SAS identifies the operating characteristics of the designs. This is not noted as being available in the paper; however, detail is given to allow implementation.

Lin and Chen (2000)

- Two-stage, multinomial outcome

- Programs noted as being available from authors

- Early termination for activity or lack of activity

Lin and Chen detail a design that considers both CRs and PRs in a trinomial outcome, weighting CR as the more desirable outcome. Investigators must specify overall response rates under the null and alternative hypotheses, and the proportion that is attributable to CR. A weighted score is calculated at the end of each stage and this is compared with predetermined cut-off boundaries as in Simon's optimal and minimax designs (to which this paper may be viewed as an extension) (Simon 1989). Tables are given for specific scenarios; however, programs are noted as being available upon request from the authors.

Panageas et al. (2002)

- Two-stage, multinomial outcome

- Programs noted as being available from authors

- Early termination for lack of activity

Panageas and colleagues propose a single-arm two-stage design based on Simon's optimal design (Simon 1989), but with a trinomial outcome (e.g. CR vs. PR vs. non-response). The design requires null and alternative response rates to be specified for both CR and PR, that is, improvements in both categories are required. The optimal design is identified iteratively, to minimise the expected sample size and to satisfy the type I and II error rates. A computer program is noted as being available from the authors, with specific design scenarios presented in tables. There is a marginal saving on sample size over Simon's design (Simon 1989). The design differs from that of Zee et al. (1999), detailed above, since early termination is permitted for lack of activity only and does not incorporate weighting of the different outcomes.

Lu et al. (2005)

- Two-stage, multinomial outcome

- Programs may be available from authors

- Early termination for lack of activity

Lu and colleagues propose a design (one-stage or two-stage) to look at both CR and total response (or other such outcome measures whereby observing one outcome implies the other outcome is also observed). The design recommends a treatment for further investigation if either of the alternative hypotheses is met (i.e. for CR or for total response) and rejects the treatment if neither is met. The designs follow the general approach of Fleming's single-stage (1982) or Simon's two-stage (Simon 1989) approach whereby the number of CRs and total responses are compared to identified stopping boundaries. Tables are provided for some combinations of null and alternative hypotheses; however, formulae are given and at the time of manuscript publication programs were in development. The design differs from others in this section in that one outcome measure is a sub-outcome measure of the other, whereas other designs consider discrete outcome measures such as PR versus CR.

Chang et al. (2007)

- Two-stage, multinomial outcome
- Programs noted as being available from authors
- Early termination for activity or lack of activity

Chang and colleagues propose a single-stage and a two-stage design for window studies which aim to assess the potential activity of a new treatment in newly diagnosed patients. Treatment is given to patients for a short period of time before standard chemotherapy, and each patient is assessed for response or early progression (both binary outcome measures). The alternative hypothesis is based on both the response rate being above a pre-specified rate *and* the early progressive disease rate being below a pre-specified rate. The outcomes follow a multinomial distribution. A SAS program is noted as being available from the authors to identify designs.

Goffin and Tu (2008)

- Two-stage, multinomial outcome
- Programs noted as being available from authors
- Early termination for lack of activity

Goffin and Tu outline an adaptation to the design proposed by Zee et al. (1999), based on a simulation approach to determine design. The authors note that the previous design of Zee was found to have lower power than intended (Freidlin et al. 2002; Zee et al. 1999). In the proposed two-stage design decision criteria are based on the proportion of patients with response and the proportion of patients with early progressive disease, in an advanced disease setting. The alternative hypothesis is that the response rate is sufficiently high or the early progressive disease rate is sufficiently low. Simulation is used to determine the required stopping boundaries to satisfy pre-specified design criteria. Programs are noted as being available upon request from the authors. Early termination is permitted for lack of activity only.

Kocherginsky et al. (2009)

- Two-stage, multinomial outcome

- Programs available from website

- Early termination for lack of activity

Kocherginsky and colleagues outline a design to consider the proportion of patients achieving response and the proportion of patients not progressing early. The alternative hypothesis being tested is that the response rate is sufficiently high or the non-progression rate is sufficiently high. Sample size is calculated via numerical searching, with the initial sample size estimate calculated following Simon's two-stage design (Simon 1989) based on the response rate limits. A numerical search is then performed over all combinations of design parameters to determine stopping rules, evaluated by assessing the probability of early termination and the probability of rejecting the null hypothesis. The design incorporates a thorough assessment of the operating characteristics over a range of response and progression rates, to guard against unexpectedly high false-positive rates under certain parameters. Programs written in R to implement the numerical search are noted as being available from http://health.bsd.uchicago.edu/filestore/biostatlab/ (last accessed July 2013). Early termination is permitted for lack of activity only.

Stallard and Cockey (2008)

- Two-stage, multinomial outcome

- Programs noted as being available from author

- Early termination for lack of activity

Stallard and Cockey propose single-arm, one- and two-stage designs for ordered categorical data, where the rejection region for the null hypothesis is defined based on the likelihood ratio test. The null region over which the type I error is controlled considers a weighting of the proportion of patients in each response category, in a similar manner to that of Lin and Chen (2000). The focus of the paper is on response with three levels; however, the design may be extended to more than three levels. Programs are noted as being available from the first author to allow identification of designs.

3.2.4   Time-to-event outcome measure

Case and Morgan (2003)

- Two-stage, time-to-event outcome

- Standard software available and programs noted as being available from authors

- Early termination for lack of activity

Case and Morgan outline a design with survival outcomes which are dichotomised to give survival probabilities at pre-specified time points of interest, incorporating all available information. The design is aimed to avoid the drawbacks of extended follow-up periods and breaks in recruitment during follow-up between stages. The design does not require a halt in recruitment between stages as Nelson–Aalen estimates of survival are used to incorporate all survival information up to the time point of interest, at the time of interim analysis. Early termination is permitted only for lack of activity. FORTRAN programs are noted as being available upon request from the authors, to identify the optimal design, and the proposed design is also available in Machin et al. (2008).

Litwin et al. (2007)

- Two-stage, time-to-event outcome
- Programs noted as being available from authors
- Early termination for activity or lack of activity

Litwin and colleagues describe a design based on the outcome measure of progression-free survival at two set time points, that is, a binary outcome. In the second stage of the design the success rate of a binary outcome measure at a set time point $t2$ is considered, which is dependent upon the success rate of a, possibly different, binary outcome measure at an earlier set time point $t1$ (assessed at the end of stage 1), for example, the progression-free rate at time $t2$, dependent upon the progression-free rate at time $t1$. The design incorporates the possibility of stopping for either activity or lack of activity at the end of the first stage and proceeds as follows:

1. $n1$ patients are recruited to the study and followed to time $t1$ for PFS.

2. If there are too few patients who are progression-free at time $t1$ then the trial is stopped early for lack of activity.

3. If there are sufficient patients who are progression-free at time $t1$ then accrual continues to the second stage until a total of $n2$ patients are recruited. Patients in the initial cohort who are progression-free at $t1$ continue on the study.

4. At the end of the second stage ($t2$) all $n2 - n1$ patients from the second stage and all those patients progression-free at $t1$ are evaluated at time $t2$.

Programs are noted as being available upon request from the authors.

3.2.5   Ratio of times to progression

No references identified.

3.3   Multi-stage designs

3.3.1   Binary outcome measure

Herson (1979)

- Multi-stage, binary outcome

- Programs noted as being available from author

- Early termination for lack of activity

Herson describes a Bayesian multi-stage design that considers early stopping rules based on the predictive probability that a treatment will not be successful at the end of the phase II trial. Early termination is therefore only permitted for lack of activity. The design incorporates investigators' prior information on the response rate of the experimental treatment and confidence in this prior information (via a coefficient of variation). Early termination boundaries are calculated based on pre-specified sample sizes ranging from 20 to 30 patients, and consideration is also given to the expected sample size of a subsequent phase III trial. Programs are noted as being available from the author.

Fleming (1982)

- Multi-stage, binary outcome

- Standard software available for overall sample size

- Early termination for activity or lack of activity

Fleming proposes a one-stage, two-stage and multi-stage design. The multi-stage design addresses multiple testing considerations to allow early termination in the case of extreme results, employing the standard single-stage test procedure at the last test. Tables are presented for specific design scenarios using the exact underlying binomial probabilities rather than the normal approximation to these probabilities. Programs are readily available to calculate the overall sample size for a one-stage design (e.g. Machin et al. 2008), with sample sizes at each stage chosen to be approximately equal. Termination at the end of each stage is permitted for activity or lack of activity.

Bellissant et al. (1990)

- Multi-stage, binary outcome

- Requires programming

- Early termination for activity or lack of activity

Bellissant and colleagues apply the triangular test (TT) and sequential probability ratio test (SPRT), previously used in phase III trials, to single-arm group-sequential phase II trials with a binary outcome. An efficient score, Z, and Fisher's information, V, are calculated derived from the likelihood function. The log odds ratio statistic is used as the measure of the difference between the actual success rate and the null hypothesis rate. Formulae are given for the calculation of Z and V as well as for calculation of the stopping boundaries, whereby Z is seen as the difference between observed and expected number of responses under the null hypothesis and V as the variance of Z under the null hypothesis. Early termination is permitted for either activity or lack of activity. Sample size is justified via the operating characteristics of the TT and SPRT, and group sizes and number of stages are arbitrary, ranging from 5 to 15 in the examples. The design requires programming to enable implementation.

Chen et al. (1994)

- Multi-stage, binary outcome

- Requires programming

- Early termination for lack of activity

Chen and colleagues propose a multi-stage design that is an extension of Gehan's two-stage design (Gehan 1961), where the chance of stopping early is increased if the observed response rate is smaller than that of interest. It is noted that this design is suitable for phase II trials that have high expected response rates, in contrast to the design of Gehan where the chance of stopping a trial early is low if the response rate of interest is above 0.3. Limited tables of designs are presented, therefore additional designs will require programming. Early termination is permitted for lack of activity only.

Ensign et al. (1994)

- Multi-stage, binary outcome

- Requires programming

- Early termination for lack of activity

Ensign and colleagues propose a single-arm three-stage design that is an extension to the two-stage design of Simon (1989). At the end of the first stage, the trial is terminated if no responses are observed (i.e. for lack of activity). If at least one response is observed, stages 2 and 3 are carried out as per Simon's stages 1 and 2. The sample sizes and cut-offs for stages 2 and 3 are determined to minimise the expected sample size under the null hypothesis. A restriction is made that the first stage must include at least five patients. Extensive tables are provided for designs under differing scenarios; however, the design will need programming to enable implementation outwith those provided.

Thall and Simon (1994a)

- Multi-stage, binary outcome

- Programs noted as being available from authors

- Early termination for lack of activity

Thall and Simon present sample size calculations for their original Bayesian continuous monitoring design (Thall and Simon 1994b). Adaptations to this design are also provided. The impact of group-sequential monitoring, as opposed to continuous monitoring, is assessed and it is found that assessment after every two, three or four patients has little impact on results; however, reducing assessments much further can increase the likelihood of inconclusive results. The first adaptation considers early stopping boundaries for inconclusive results. The second adaptation considers early termination for lack of activity, which considers only lower stopping boundaries. Software is noted as being available upon request to compute and implement each of these designs, including the original continuous monitoring design (Thall and Simon 1994b).

Tan and Xiong (1996)

- Multi-stage, binary outcome

- Programs available on website

- Early termination for activity or lack of activity

Tan and Xiong propose a group-sequential (or continuous monitoring) design for the assessment of a binary outcome in a single-arm trial, based on the sequential conditional probability ratio test (SCPRT). The design is based around comparison to a reference fixed sample size test (RFSST) such as that proposed by Fleming (1982), and the results that this would achieve, since it is desirable to preserve the power of this test while incorporating additional opportunities to terminate the trial early. The proposed design provides similar power to the fixed sample size test, but allows more opportunity to terminate the trial early (for activity or lack of activity). A FORTRAN program is available via the website (http://lib.stat.cmu.edu/designs/scprtbin (last accessed July 2013)) to compute the design characteristics.

Chen (1997)

- Multi-stage, binary outcome

- Program noted as being available from author

- Early termination for lack of activity

Chen proposes an extension to Simon's minimax and optimal two-stage designs (Simon 1989), simply incorporating an additional stage. Tables are provided with designs under various scenarios, and a FORTRAN program is noted as being available from the author for other scenarios. When compared to Simon's design, the three-stage design sometimes has smaller expected sample size; however, this is not consistent. Compared to Ensign's three-stage design (Ensign et al. 1994), the proposed design does not make restrictions on the size and cut-off for the first stage.

Murray et al. (2004)

- Multi-stage, binary outcome
- Requires programming
- Early termination for activity or lack of activity

Murray and colleagues detail calculation of stopping rules based on confidence interval estimation of the response rate at each stage. A table of specific design scenarios is presented; however, the design requires programming to identify optimal decision criteria for scenarios outwith the tables. The design is based on a pre-specified fixed sample size (i.e. no sample size calculation is performed) and a fixed number of stages (with fixed sample size at each stage), with type I and II errors evaluated for the resulting design. Early termination is permitted for either activity or lack of activity. The design may be used when only a small number of patients are available for study (30 patients considered in the motivating example) and exact binomial calculations are employed.

Ayanlowo and Redden (2007)

- Multi-stage, binary outcome
- Requires programming
- Early termination for lack of activity

Ayanlowo and Redden propose a stochastic curtailment design which is based on the simple binomial test and considers the conditional probability of declaring a treatment active at the end of the trial, conditional upon the responses observed to date and the assumption that the alternative hypothesis is true. The design requires programming to identify the points at which to conduct interim assessments. Sample size determination is based on a binomial test. Stochastic curtailment adaptations to Simon's minimax and optimal design are also proposed (Simon 1989). While the proposed designs provide more opportunity to stop a trial early due to an inactive treatment, the authors suggest its use only when Simon's minimax design is already being considered, and when the trial is expected to recruit slowly and the outcome may be observed relatively quickly.

Chen and Shan (2008)

- Multi-stage, binary outcome
- Programs noted as being available from authors
- Early termination for activity or lack of activity

Chen and Shan outline a three-stage design, extending previous designs to allow early termination for either activity or lack of activity (Chen 1997; Ensign et al. 1994; Simon 1989). Tables are given for optimal and minimax designs where the difference in null and alternative hypothesis rates is 0.20 or 0.15, for a number of scenarios. A C program is noted as being available from the authors to search for designs under alternative scenarios. Comparing the proposed optimal and minimax designs with those of Chen (1997), the designs presented in the current paper require larger maximal sample size under the optimal design and similar maximal sample size under the minimax design, but have a smaller average sample number in most cases. Due to the ability to terminate early for either activity or lack of activity, the probability of early termination at the first stage and overall is higher for the current designs compared to those of Chen (1997).

Lee and Liu (2008)

- Multi-stage, binary outcome

- Programs available from website

- Early termination for lack of activity or activity

Lee and Liu outline a Bayesian group-sequential/continuous monitoring design based on a binary outcome and the use of predictive probabilities (probability of a positive result should the trial run to conclusion, given the interim data observed). The design incorporates early termination for lack of activity, as well as activity. The continuous monitoring design is compared to Simon's two-stage design (Simon 1989). Under the proposed approach the probability of stopping the trial early is higher, and in general, the expected sample size under the null hypothesis is smaller. When assessing the design for robustness to deviation from continuous monitoring, although the type I error rate is inflated (usually less than 10%) the design generally remains robust. The authors provide further considerations of robustness to early termination, estimation bias and comparison to posterior probability designs. Software is available from https://biostatistics.mdanderson.org/Software Download/SingleSoftware.aspx?Software_Id=84 (last accessed July 2013) to allow implementation.

3.3.2   Continuous outcome measure

No references identified.

3.3.3   Multinomial outcome measure

Zee et al. (1999)

- Multi-stage, multinomial outcome

- Requires programming

- Early termination for activity or lack of activity

Zee and colleagues propose single-stage and multi-stage single-arm designs considering a multinomial outcome, in the context of incorporating progressive disease as well as response into the primary outcome measure. Analysis is based on the number of responses and progressions observed, compared with predetermined stopping criteria. A computer program written in SAS identifies the operating characteristics of the designs. This is not noted as being available in the paper; however, detail is given to allow implementation.

3.3.4   Time-to-event outcome measure

Cheung and Thall (2002)

- Multi-stage, time-to-event outcome

- Programs noted as being available from authors

- Early termination for activity or lack of activity

Cheung and Thall propose a Bayesian sequential-adaptive procedure for continuous monitoring, which may be extended to assessment after cohorts of more than one patient, that is, multi-stage. The outcome measure of interest is a binary indicator of a composite time-to-event outcome, utilising all the censored and uncensored observations at each interim assessment. Continuous monitoring based on the approximate posterior (CMAP) is used following Thall and Simon (1994b). The design can incorporate multiple competing and non-competing outcomes. Early termination is permitted for activity or lack of activity. R programs are noted as being available from the authors to allow implementation of the design. This design enables data to be incorporated on all patients at each interim assessment without all follow-up data being obtained and may therefore be used when follow-up of each patient is for a non-trivial period of time.

3.3.5   Ratio of times to progression

No references identified.

3.4   Continuous monitoring designs

3.4.1   Binary outcome measure

Thall and Simon (1994b)

- Continuous monitoring, binary outcome

- Programs noted as being available from authors

- Early termination for activity or lack of activity

Thall and Simon propose a Bayesian continuous monitoring design to assess the binary outcome of response in a single-arm trial. Information required includes prior information on the standard treatment, required improvement due to the experimental treatment and minimum and maximum boundaries on sample size. A flat prior is assumed for the experimental treatment. Also required is a concentration parameter for the experimental treatment, representing the amount of dispersion about the mean of the experimental treatment. After the response outcome is observed on each patient, the trial may be terminated for lack of activity, terminated for activity or continued to the next patient (although this assessment is not required before the next patient can be recruited). If the maximum sample size is obtained and neither of the stopping boundaries for activity or lack of activity is crossed, the trial is declared inconclusive. Stopping boundaries are calculated in terms of upper and lower posterior probability limits, calculated by numerical integration. Designs should be assessed by simulation to investigate the operating characteristics. Detail regarding software and implementation is presented elsewhere (Thall and Simon 1994a).

Thall and Simon (1994a)

- Continuous monitoring, binary outcome

- Programs noted as being available from authors

- Early termination for lack of activity

Thall and Simon present sample size calculations for their original Bayesian continuous monitoring design (Thall and Simon 1994b) outlined above. Adaptations to this design are also provided. The first adaptation considers early stopping boundaries for inconclusive results. The second adaptation considers early termination for lack of activity, which considers only lower stopping boundaries. Software is noted as being available upon request to compute and implement the designs, including the original continuous monitoring design (Thall and Simon 1994b).

Tan and Xiong (1996)

- Continuous monitoring, binary outcome

- Programs available on website

- Early termination for activity or lack of activity

Tan and Xiong propose a group-sequential (or continuous monitoring) design for the assessment of a binary outcome in a single-arm trial, based on the SCPRT. The design is based around comparison to a RFSST such as that proposed by Fleming (1982), and the results that this would achieve, since it is desirable to preserve the power of this test while incorporating additional opportunities to terminate the trial early. The proposed design provides similar power to the fixed sample size test, but allows more opportunity to terminate the trial early (for activity or lack of activity). A FORTRAN program is available via the website (http://lib.stat.cmu.edu/designs/scprtbin (last accessed July 2013)) to compute the design characteristics.

Chen and Chaloner (2006)

- Continuous monitoring, binary outcome

- Programs noted as being available from authors

- Early termination for lack of activity

Chen and Chaloner propose a stopping rule for a Bayesian continuous monitoring design. Stopping rules are based on both the posterior probability that the failure rate is unacceptably high and the posterior probability that the failure rate is acceptably low, where these high and low values are derived from historical data. Patients are recruited until either the stopping rules are met or a maximum sample size has been recruited. Programs are noted as being available in R (via contacting the authors) to enable computation of the stopping boundaries and operating characteristics based on maximum sample size available, prior information on the experimental treatment, null and alternative hypothesis rates and the upper and lower posterior probability bounds. Early termination is permitted only for lack of activity.

Lee and Liu (2008)

- Continuous monitoring, binary outcome

- Programs available from website

- Early termination for lack of activity or activity

Lee and Liu outline a Bayesian group-sequential/continuous monitoring design based on a binary outcome and the use of predictive probabilities (probability of a positive result should the trial run to conclusion, given the interim data observed). The design incorporates early termination for lack of activity, as well as activity. The continuous monitoring design is compared to Simon's two-stage design (Simon 1989). Under the proposed approach the probability of stopping the trial early is higher, and in general, the expected sample size under the null hypothesis is smaller. When assessing the design for robustness to deviation from continuous monitoring, although the type I error rate is inflated (usually less than 10%) the design generally remains robust. The authors provide further considerations of robustness to early termination, estimation bias and comparison to posterior probability designs. Software is available from https://biostatistics.mdanderson.org/Software Download/SingleSoftware.aspx?Software_Id=84 (last accessed July 2013) to allow implementation.

Johnson and Cook (2009)

- Continuous monitoring, binary outcome

- Programs available on website

- Early termination for lack of activity or activity

Johnson and Cook propose a Bayesian continuous monitoring design based on formal hypothesis tests. They argue that, in contrast to Bayesian designs based on posterior credible intervals, any misspecification of prior densities associated with the alternative hypothesis cannot bias the trial results in favour of the null hypothesis when the proposed formal hypothesis test approach is used. Analysis is performed after data are available for each patient, and the trial may be terminated early for activity or lack of activity. Software is available from https://bio statistics.mdanderson.org/SoftwareDownload/SingleSoftware.aspx?Software_Id=94 (last accessed July 2013) which allows the trial to be designed according to user-specified priors.

3.4.2 Continuous outcome measure

No references identified.

3.4.3 Multinomial outcome measure

No references identified.

3.4.4 Time-to-event outcome measure

Cheung and Thall (2002)

- Continuous monitoring, time-to-event outcome

- Programs noted as being available from authors

- Early termination for activity or lack of activity

Cheung and Thall propose a Bayesian sequential-adaptive procedure for continuous monitoring. The outcome measure of interest is a binary indicator of a composite time-to-event outcome, utilising all the censored and uncensored observations at each interim assessment. Continuous monitoring based on the approximate posterior (CMAP) is used following Thall and Simon (1994b). The design can incorporate multiple competing and non-competing outcomes. Early termination is permitted for activity or lack of activity. R programs are noted as being available from the author to allow implementation of the design. This design enables data to be incorporated on all patients at each assessment without all follow-up data being obtained and may therefore be used when follow-up of each patient is for a non-trivial period of time.

Thall et al. (2005)

- Continuous monitoring, time-to-event outcome

- Programs noted as being available from authors

- Early termination for activity or lack of activity

Thall and colleagues propose Bayesian continuous monitoring designs that incorporate three time-to-event outcomes (death, disease progression and SAE). Various amendments to the design are proposed, including randomisation, frequent interval monitoring, alternative distribution assumptions and incorporation of interval censoring for disease progression. The trial may be stopped early for lack of activity or for activity. Simulations are performed to establish operating characteristics of the designs. Programs are noted as being available from the authors upon request.

Johnson and Cook (2009)

- Continuous monitoring, time-to-event outcome

- Programs available on website

- Early termination for lack of activity or activity

Johnson and Cook propose a Bayesian continuous monitoring design based on formal hypothesis tests. They argue that, in contrast to Bayesian designs based on posterior credible intervals, any misspecification of prior densities associated with the alternative hypothesis cannot bias the trial results in favour of the null hypothesis when the proposed formal hypothesis test approach is used. Analysis is performed after data are available for each patient, and the trial may be terminated early for activity or lack of activity. Software is available from https://bio statistics.mdanderson.org/SoftwareDownload/SingleSoftware.aspx?Software_Id=94 (last accessed July 2013) which allows the trial to be designed according to user-specified priors.

3.4.5   Ratio of times to progression

No references identified.

3.5   Decision-theoretic designs

3.5.1   Binary outcome measure

Sylvester and Staquet (1980)

- Decision-theoretic, binary outcome

- Requires programming

- Early termination for activity or lack of activity

Sylvester and Staquet outline a decision-theoretic design whereby the sample size and cut-off boundaries for decision-making in the phase II trial are calculated based on the number of patients who would be expected to receive the experimental treatment in a subsequent phase III trial, as well as prior probabilities of the response proportions of the experimental treatment in the phase II trial. There are examples of specific design scenarios; however, the design would require programming to enable implementation. Decision criteria are based on observing a given number of responses. The design allows incorporation of interim assessments, at which the trial may be terminated early for either activity or lack of activity.

3.5.2   Continuous outcome measure

No references identified.

3.5.3   Multinomial outcome measure

No references identified.

3.5.4   Time-to-event outcome measure

No references identified.

3.5.5   Ratio of times to progression

No references identified.

3.6   Three-outcome designs

3.6.1   Binary outcome measure

Lee et al. (1979)

- Three-outcome design, binary outcome
- Requires programming
- Early termination for activity or lack of activity

Lee and colleagues present a two-stage, three-outcome design whereby the available sample size is pre-specified based on non-statistical considerations such as patient availability, and the optimal design is identified based on given constraints. The design is based on determining whether the true response rate is above or below a single pre-specified response rate, incorporating the possibility to declare an inconclusive result. Tables are presented for a target 20% response rate only, with upper and lower limits of 30% and 10%, respectively, for determining activity, lack of activity or an inconclusive result. The paper is therefore somewhat impractical for designs beyond this specific setting, without further work to implement for other scenarios. The design may be seen to complement the confidence interval approach to estimating a response rate with given precision.

Storer (1992)

- Three-outcome design, binary outcome
- Programs noted as being available from author
- Early termination for activity or lack of activity

Storer proposes a three-outcome design that is an adaptation to single-, two- and multi-stage designs such as those described by Fleming (1982). The event rate of uncertainty is taken to be around the midpoint between the event rate of no interest and the event rate of interest. As described in Chapter 2, various error rates are required to be specified. Here the probabilities of concluding in favour of either the null or alternative hypothesis when in fact the true response rate lies within the region of uncertainty are required to be specified. These error rates are set to be equal under this design. Programs are noted as being available to identify the design, upon request from the author. Early termination is permitted for activity or lack of activity in the two- and multi-stage designs.

Sargent et al. (2001)

- Three-outcome design, binary outcome
- Requires programming; programs may be available upon request
- Early termination for lack of activity

Sargent and colleagues propose a single-stage (and two-stage) design with three possible outcomes. As described in Chapter 2, various error rates are required to be specified, corresponding to differing regions of the distribution curves presented in Figure 2.2. Here specific probabilities for concluding uncertainty are specified under both the null and alternative hypotheses (λ and δ, respectively, in Figure 2.2), and these may differ. Tables and formulae are provided for sample size and stopping rule calculation. The design requires programming; however, programs may be available upon request from the authors. Under the two-stage design, early termination is for lack of activity only.

3.6.2   Continuous outcome measure

No references identified.

3.6.3   Multinomial outcome measure

No references identified.

3.6.4   Time-to-event outcome measure

No references identified.

3.6.5   Ratio of times to progression

No references identified.

3.7   Phase II/III designs

There are no phase II/III designs listed in this chapter since these designs require a control arm to be incorporated in the phase II trial, to enable a seamless transition to phase III.

4

Designs for single experimental therapies including randomisation

Sarah Brown

The designs included in this chapter incorporate randomisation to a control arm with the intention of a formally powered statistical comparison between the experimental and control arms, as well as designs where incorporation of randomisation is primarily to provide a calibration arm, with no statistical comparison formally powered. The distinction between these approaches is presented for each design listed.

4.1   One-stage designs

4.1.1   Binary outcome measure

Herson and Carter (1986)

- One-stage, binary outcome

- No formally powered statistical comparison between arms

- Requires programming

Herson and Carter consider the inclusion of a randomised calibration group in single-stage phase II trials of a binary endpoint, in order to reduce the risk of

A Practical Guide to Designing Phase II Trials in Oncology, First Edition.
Sarah R. Brown, Walter M. Gregory, Chris Twelves and Julia Brown.
© 2014 John Wiley & Sons, Ltd. Published 2014 by John Wiley & Sons, Ltd.

false-negative decision-making. Patients are randomised between current standard treatment (calibration group) and the treatment under investigation. Results of the calibration group are intended largely to assess the credibility of the outcome in the experimental arm, that is, not for formal comparative purposes. Decision criteria are based primarily on the experimental arm results; however, outcomes in the calibration arm are also considered to address the initial assumptions made regarding the current standard treatment. Thus the trial essentially constitutes two separate designs, one for the experimental arm and one for the calibration arm. Due to the assessment of the control arm results, the overall sample size of the trial may be between three and five times that of a non-calibrated design. An example is provided; however, the design will require programming.

Thall and Simon (1990)

- One-stage, binary outcome

- No formally powered statistical comparison between arms

- Requires programming

Thall and Simon outline a design that incorporates historical data, including variability, into the design of the trial. A specific proportion of patients are randomised to a control arm dependent upon the amount of historical control data available, the degree of both inter-study and intra-study variability and the overall sample size of the phase II study being planned (following formulae provided). The inclusion of a sample of patients randomised to a control arm allows the precision of the response rate in the experimental arm at the end of the trial to be maximised, relative to the control. Sample size is determined iteratively and the design would need to be programmed to allow implementation.

Stone et al. (2007b)

- One-stage, binary outcome

- Formally powered statistical comparison between arms

- Standard software available

Stone et al. discuss the use of progressive disease rate at a given time point (as well as overall progression-free survival) as an outcome measure in randomised phase II trials of cytostatic agents. Formal comparison between the experimental treatment and the control treatment is performed for superiority; however, larger type I error rates than would be used in phase III are incorporated, and large treatment effects are targeted. The use of relaxed type I errors and large targeted treatment effects contribute to reduced sample sizes compared to phase III trials, and may therefore be deemed more realistic for phase II trials.

4.1.2   Continuous outcome measure

Thall and Simon (1990)

- One-stage, continuous outcome

- No formally powered statistical comparison between arms

- Requires programming

Thall and Simon outline a design that incorporates historical data, including variability, into the design of the trial. A specific proportion of patients are randomised to a control arm dependent upon the amount of historical control data available, the degree of both inter-study and intra-study variability and the overall sample size of the phase II study being planned (following formulae provided). The inclusion of a sample of patients randomised to a control arm allows the precision of the outcome estimate in the experimental arm at the end of the trial to be maximised, relative to the control. Sample size is determined iteratively and the design would need to be programmed to allow implementation.

Chen and Beckman (2009)

- One-stage, continuous outcome

- Formally powered statistical comparison between arms

- Programming code provided

Chen and Beckman describe an approach to a randomised phase II trial design that incorporates optimal error rates. Optimal type I and II errors for the design are identified by means of an efficiency score function which is based on initial proposed error rates and the ratio of sample sizes between phases II and III. Sample size calculation is performed using standard phase III-type approaches using the optimal identified type I and II errors. Formal comparison with the control arm is incorporated. The design considers cost efficiency of the phase II and III trials, on the basis of the ratio of sample sizes between phases II and III and the *a priori* probability of success of the investigational treatment. An R program is provided in the appendix of the manuscript to identify optimal designs.

4.1.3   Multinomial outcome measure

No references identified.

4.1.4   Time-to-event outcome measure

Simon et al. (2001)

- One-stage, time-to-event outcome

- Formally powered statistical comparison between arms

- Standard software available

Simon and colleagues propose what is termed a randomised 'phase 2.5' trial design, incorporating intermediate outcome measures such as progression-free survival. The design takes the approach of a phase III trial design, with a formally powered statistical comparison with the control arm for superiority. It incorporates a relaxed significance level, large targeted treatment effects and intermediate outcome measures, resulting in more pragmatic and feasible sample sizes than would be required in a phase III trial. The design is straightforward, following the methodology of phase III trials; however, it is important to note that this should only be used where large treatment differences are realistic and should not be seen as a way to eliminate phase III testing.

Stone et al. (2007b)

- One-stage, time-to-event outcome

- Formally powered statistical comparison between arms

- Standard software available

Stone et al. discuss the use of progressive disease rate at a given time point, as well as overall progression-free survival, as an outcome measure in randomised phase II trials of cytostatic agents. Formal comparison between the experimental treatment and the control treatment is performed for superiority; however, larger type I error rates than would be used in phase III are incorporated, and large treatment effects are targeted. The use of relaxed type I errors and large targeted treatment effects contribute to reduced sample sizes compared to phase III trials, and may therefore be deemed more realistic for phase II trials. This reflects the designs described above by Simon et al. in the setting of time-to-event outcomes, which are described by the authors as 'phase 2.5' designs (Simon et al. 2001).

Chen and Beckman (2009)

- One-stage, time-to-event outcome

- Formally powered statistical comparison between arms

- Programming code provided

Chen and Beckman describe an approach to a randomised phase II trial design that incorporates optimal error rates. Optimal type I and II errors for the design are identified by means of an efficiency score function which is based on initial proposed error rates and the ratio of sample sizes between phases II and III. Sample size calculation is performed using standard phase III-type approaches using the optimal identified type I and II errors. Formal comparison with the control arm is incorporated. The design considers cost efficiency of the phase II and III trials, on the basis of the ratio of sample sizes between phases II and III and the *a priori* probability of success of the investigational treatment. An R program is provided in the appendix of the manuscript to identify optimal designs.

4.1.5   Ratio of times to progression

No references identified.

4.2   Two-stage designs

4.2.1   Binary outcome measure

Whitehead et al. (2009)

- Two-stage, binary outcome
- Formally powered statistical comparison between arms
- Requires programming
- Early termination for activity or lack of activity

Whitehead and colleagues outline a randomised controlled two-stage design with normally distributed outcome measures that may be extended to the setting of binary and ordinal outcomes. The design allows early termination for activity, or lack of activity, and incorporates formal comparison between experimental and control arms. At the interim assessment, which takes place after approximately half the total number of patients have been recruited, sample size re-estimation may be incorporated if necessary. The methodology employs approximations to the normal distribution since sample sizes are generally large enough. No software is detailed as being available to identify designs; however, programming is noted as being possible in SAS, and detail is provided to allow its implementation. Simulation is also required to evaluate potential designs.

Jung (2008)

- Two-stage, binary outcome
- Formally powered statistical comparison between arms
- Programs noted as being available from author
- Early termination for lack of activity

Jung proposes a randomised controlled extension to Simon's optimal and minimax designs (Simon 1989) in the context of a binary outcome measure (e.g. response). The experimental arm is formally compared with the control arm and declared worthy of further investigation only if there are sufficiently more responders in the experimental arm. Extensive tables are provided, and programs to identify designs not included in tables are noted as being available upon request from the author. Extensions to the design include unequal allocation, strict type I and II error control and randomisation to more than one experimental arm.

Jung and George (2009)

- Two-stage, binary outcome

- Formally powered statistical comparison between arms

- Requires minimal programming

- Early termination for lack of efficacy

Jung and George propose methods of comparing treatment arms in a randomised phase II trial, where the intention is either to determine whether a single treatment is worthy of evaluation compared to a control or to select one treatment from many for further evaluation. The phase II design for a single experimental treatment versus control is initially based on the evaluation of the control and experimental arms independently following Simon's two-stage design (Simon 1989), or similar. The experimental treatment must first be accepted via this evaluation, that is, compared to historical control rates, and is then formally compared with the concurrent control arm. The experimental treatment is deemed worthy of further evaluation if the treatment difference between the two arms is above some pre-defined value. No software is detailed; however, detail is given which should allow implementation, and sufficient examples are also provided. The initial two-stage design can be calculated using standard software available for Simon's two-stage design.

4.2.2   Continuous outcome measure

Whitehead et al. (2009)

- Two-stage, continuous outcome

- Formally powered statistical comparison between arms

- Requires programming

- Early termination for activity or lack of activity

Whitehead and colleagues outline a randomised controlled two-stage design with normally distributed outcome measures. The design allows early termination for activity, or lack of activity, and incorporates formal comparison between experimental and control arms. At the interim assessment, which takes place after approximately half the total number of patients have been recruited, sample size re-estimation may be incorporated if necessary. The methodology employs approximations to the normal distribution since sample sizes are generally large enough. No software is detailed as being available to identify designs; however, programming is noted as being possible in SAS, and detail is provided to allow its implementation. Simulation is also required to evaluate potential designs. The authors note that the design may be extended to binary and ordinal outcome measures.

4.2.3   Multinomial outcome measure

Whitehead et al. (2009)

- Two-stage, multinomial outcome
- Formally powered statistical comparison between arms
- Requires programming
- Early termination for activity or lack of activity

Whitehead and colleagues outline a randomised controlled two-stage design with normally distributed outcome measures, which may be extended to binary and ordinal outcome measures. The design allows early termination for activity, and lack of activity, and incorporates formal comparison between experimental and control arms. At the interim assessment, which takes place after approximately half the total number of patients have been recruited, sample size re-estimation may be incorporated if necessary. The methodology employs approximations to the normal distribution since sample sizes are generally large enough. No software is detailed as being available to identify designs; however, programming is noted as being possible in SAS, and detail is provided to allow its implementation. Simulation is also required to evaluate potential designs.

Sun et al. (2009)

- Two-stage, multinomial outcome
- Formally powered statistical comparison between arms
- Software noted as being available from author
- Early termination for lack of activity

Sun and colleagues propose a randomised two-stage design based on Zee's single-arm multi-stage design with multinomial outcome measure (Zee et al. 1999), adjusting the rules such that a sufficiently high response rate *or* a sufficiently low early progressive disease rate should warrant further investigation of the treatment. Optimal and minimax designs are proposed following the methodology of Simon (1989). Differences in response and progressive disease rates between control and experimental arms are compared, and the authors note that the intention of the phase II trial is to screen for potential efficacy as opposed to identifying statistically significant differences. An extension is also proposed to the multi-arm selection setting. Detail is given regarding how to implement the designs in practice, and software is noted as being available by contacting the first author to allow identification of designs. The design recommends a treatment for further investigation when the response rate is sufficiently high, or the early progressive disease rate is sufficiently low. Early termination is permitted for lack of activity only. The authors also note that the design may be extended to studies monitoring safety and efficacy simultaneously.

4.2.4   Time-to-event outcome measure

No references identified.

4.2.5   Ratio of times to progression

No references identified.

4.3   Multi-stage designs

4.3.1   Binary outcome measure

No references identified.

4.3.2   Continuous outcome measure

Cronin et al. (1999)

- Multi-stage, continuous outcome

- Formally powered statistical comparison between arms

- Standard software available for sample size

- Early termination for activity or lack of activity

Cronin and colleagues propose a Bayesian design for monitoring of phase II trials. The design incorporates both sceptical and indifferent priors at each of the interim analyses, according to the hypothesis being tested. Early termination is permitted for activity or lack of activity, and as such, priors differ at interim and final analysis. Posterior distributions are updated at each analysis. When compared with frequentist group-sequential methods, the proposed Bayesian methods performed at least as well for the main purpose of detecting ineffective treatments early. The Bayesian method was slowest to stop when the treatment had clear biological activity. The authors note that the Bayesian method provides flexibility to make changes to outcome measures, analyses and original trial plans at interim analyses without introducing theoretical statistical complications. Standard software is available for sample size calculation.

4.3.3   Multinomial outcome measure

No references identified.

4.3.4   Time-to-event outcome measure

No references identified.

4.3.5   Ratio of times to progression

No references identified.

4.4   Continuous monitoring designs

4.4.1   Binary outcome measure

No references identified.

4.4.2   Continuous outcome measure

No references identified.

4.4.3   Multinomial outcome measure

No references identified.

4.4.4   Time-to-event outcome measure

Thall et al. (2005)

- Continuous monitoring, time-to-event outcome
- Formally powered statistical comparison between arms
- Programs available from authors
- Early termination for activity or lack of activity

Thall and colleagues propose Bayesian continuous monitoring designs that incorporate three time-to-event outcomes (death, disease progression and serious adverse event). Various amendments to the initial proposed single-arm continuous monitoring design assuming exponential distribution are proposed (Cheung and Thall 2002), including randomisation, frequent interval monitoring, alternative distribution assumptions and incorporation of interval censoring for disease progression. The trial may be stopped early for lack of activity or for activity. Simulations are performed to assess the performance of the design. Programs are noted as being available from the authors upon request.

4.4.5   Ratio of times to progression

No references identified.

4.5   Three-outcome designs

4.5.1   Binary outcome measure

Hong and Wang (2007)

- Three-outcome design, binary outcome measure

- Formally powered statistical comparison between arms

- Programs noted as being available from authors

- Early termination for lack of activity

Hong and Wang detail both a single-stage and a two-stage three-outcome design which extend that of Sargent et al. (2001) (Chapter 3) to a randomised comparative design. The region of uncertainty falls around the middle region between the null hypothesis that the difference in response rates between the arms is zero and the alternative hypothesis that the difference is delta. In the two-stage design the trial may only be terminated at the end of the first stage for lack of activity. A SAS program to identify the design is noted as being available on request from the authors.

4.5.2   Continuous outcome measure

No references identified.

4.5.3   Multinomial outcome measure

No references identified.

4.5.4   Time-to-event outcome measure

No references identified.

4.5.5   Ratio of times to progression

No references identified.

4.6   Phase II/III designs

4.6.1   Binary outcome measure

Storer (1990)

- Phase II/III, binary outcome

- No formal comparison with control in phase II

- Standard software available for phase II, phase III requires programming

- No early termination during phase II

Storer proposes a phase II/III design with the same binary outcome at both stages. This corresponds to a single-arm phase II design (e.g. A'Hern 2001) embedded in a randomised phase III trial (i.e. randomisation takes place in phase II but the design and primary decision-making are based on a single-arm design). The phase II decision criteria are based on the results of the experimental arm only, as opposed to comparing activity between the experimental and control arms. Sample size calculations for the phase II aspect may be performed using standard available software for one-stage designs, based on numerical searching to satisfy given type I and II errors and null and alternative hypothesis response rates. Standard approaches to phase III sample size calculation are used, with formulae provided to incorporate an adjustment for the phase II/III design. This design may be used as a basis for phase II/III designs whereby any single-arm phase II design is embedded in a phase III trial, including where the outcome measure at phase III differs to that at phase II.

The design described above uses the same outcome measure at phase II as it does at phase III. Although this may be seen as seamless phase II/III approach, in effect it reflects a phase III trial with an early interim analysis on the primary outcome measure (albeit based on a single-arm design). In this setting, consideration should be given to the most appropriate outcome measure to use for both the phase II *and* phase III primary outcome. It is rare that efficacy in the phase III setting could be claimed on the basis of a binary outcome; rather, a time-to-event outcome is usually required in phase III trials.

Lachin and Younes (2007)

- Phase II/III, binary outcome

- Formally powered statistical comparison between arms

- Requires programming

- No early termination during phase II

Lachin and Younes outline a phase II/III design that incorporates different outcome measures at phases II and III (with phase II being a shorter term outcome measure). Joint distributions for the phase II and III outcomes are calculated, and the design operating characteristics and sample sizes are calculated via iteration and numerical integration. An estimate of the correlation between the two outcome measures is required. The design preserves the type I and II error rates, and patients randomised during phase II are included in the phase III analysis. Analysis of the phase II outcome measure considers a formal comparison for lack of activity only (or excessive toxicity). Software is not detailed as being available; therefore, this design would require programming to allow implementation.

Chow and Tu (2008)

- Phase II/III, binary outcome

- Formally powered statistical comparison between arms

- Requires programming

- No early termination during phase II

Chow and Tu present sample size formulae for seamless adaptive phase II/III designs where the outcome measures at each phase differ, but the outcome measure distributions remain the same (e.g. binary outcome in phase II, binary outcome in phase III). This design is based on two separate studies, with differing endpoints and durations, which are then combined. Data from patients in the phase II trial are used to predict the phase III endpoint, for those patients, rather than continuing to follow patients to observe the phase III endpoint. These data are then combined with the data from the phase III trial. The relationship between the outcome measures at each phase is required to be known and well established. This is an essential component due to the predictive nature of the design. The design will require programming to enable implementation.

4.6.2   Continuous outcome measure

Liu and Pledger (2005)

- Phase II/III, continuous outcome

- Formally powered statistical comparison between arms

- Requires programming

- No early termination during phase II

Liu and Pledger detail a phase II/III design for a single experimental treat-ment compared to a control, as well as outlining a design in the dose-finding context. In the single experimental treatment setting, the experimental treatment is compared with the control treatment at the end of the phase II trial, based on the short-term continuous outcome measure associated with the phase II trial. At this stage, there is no break in recruitment during the analysis, and the sample size for the phase III trial may be modified to allow estimation of the standard deviation of the phase III outcome measure. Different phase II and III outcome measures are used. At the end of the trial, the test statistics from the first and sec-ond stages (i.e. phases II and III) are combined. The treatment effect required to be observed is the same for both short- and long-term outcome measures and needs to be pre-specified, along with prior information on probability of success and stan-dard deviation for each outcome measure. This information is used to generate the operating characteristics of the design. Formulae are given which would need to be implemented in order to identify the design. The design offers flexibility in that the second-stage (phase III) sample size may be calculated based on updated data from the first stage (phase II), and adaptation rules do not need to be specified in advance.

Lachin and Younes (2007)

- Phase II/III, continuous outcome

- Formally powered statistical comparison between arms

- Requires programming

- No early termination during phase II

Lachin and Younes outline a phase II/III design that incorporates different outcome measures at phases II and III (with phase II being a shorter term outcome measure). Joint distributions for the phase II and III outcomes are calculated, and the design operating characteristics and sample sizes are calculated via iteration and numerical integration. An estimate of the correlation between the two outcome measures is required. The design preserves the type I and II error rates, and patients randomised during phase II are included in the phase III analysis. Analysis of the phase II outcome measure considers a formal comparison for lack of activity only (or excessive toxicity). Software is not detailed as being available; therefore, this design would require programming to allow implementation. Detail is provided for binary and continuous phase II outcome measures; however, extensions to time-to-event outcomes are discussed.

Chow and Tu (2008)

- Phase II/III, continuous outcome

- Formally powered statistical comparison between arms

- Requires programming

- No early termination in phase II

Chow and Tu present sample size formulae for seamless adaptive phase II/III designs where the outcome measures at each phase differ, but the outcome measure distributions remain the same (e.g. binary outcome in phase II, binary outcome in phase III). This design is based on two separate studies, with differing endpoints and durations, which are then combined. Data from patients in the phase II trial are used to predict the phase III endpoint, for those patients, rather than continuing to follow patients to observe the phase III endpoint. These data are then combined with the data from the phase III trial. The relationship between the outcome measures at each phase is required to be known and well established. This is an essential component due to the predictive nature of the design. The design will require programming to enable implementation.

4.6.3   Multinomial outcome measure

No references identified.

4.6.4   Time-to-event outcome measure

Lachin and Younes (2007)

- Phase II/III, time-to-event outcome

- Formally powered statistical comparison between arms

- Requires programming

- No early termination during phase II

Lachin and Younes outline a phase II/III design that incorporates different outcome measures at phases II and III (with phase II being a shorter term outcome measure). Joint distributions for the phase II and III outcomes are calculated, and the design operating characteristics and sample sizes are calculated via iteration and numerical integration. An estimate of the correlation between the two outcome measures is required. The design preserves the type I and II error rates, and patients randomised during phase II are included in the phase III analysis. Analysis of the phase II outcome measure considers a formal comparison for lack of activity only (or excessive toxicity). Software is not detailed as being available; therefore, this design would require programming to allow implementation.

Chow and Tu (2008)

- Phase II/III, time-to-event outcome

- Formally powered statistical comparison between arms

- Requires programming

- No early termination in phase II

Chow and Tu present sample size formulae for seamless adaptive phase II/III designs where the outcome measures at each phase differ, but the outcome measure distributions remain the same (e.g. binary outcome in phase II, binary outcome in phase III). This design is based on two separate studies, with differing endpoints and durations, which are then combined. Data from patients in the phase II trial are used to predict the phase III endpoint, for those patients, rather than continuing to follow patients to observe the phase III endpoint. These data are then combined with the data from the phase III trial. The relationship between the outcome measures at each phase is required to be known and well established. This is an essential component due to the predictive nature of the design. The design will require programming to enable implementation.

4.6.5   Ratio of times to progression

No references identified.

4.7   Randomised discontinuation designs

4.7.1   Binary outcome measure

Kopec et al. (1993)

- Randomised discontinuation, binary outcome

- Formally powered statistical comparison between arms

- Requires programming (can incorporate standard software)

- No early termination

Kopec et al. introduce the randomised discontinuation design. All eligible patients are initially treated with the investigational treatment for a pre-defined period of time. At this time, all patients are assessed for response to treatment. Treatment 'responders' are randomised to either continue with the investigational treatment or to discontinue the investigational treatment (and instead receive a placebo or current standard treatment). A formal comparison is made between the experimental and control arms at the end of the second stage (i.e. after randomisation). Formulae for the calculation of response proportions are provided and are based on the sample size needed for the randomised phase to assess relative activity. The design would therefore need programming. Analysis may also be adapted to incorporate data from patients in the first stage, to adapt the response requirements for randomisation, for example, to incorporate patients with stable disease or greater, as detailed by Rosner et al. (2002). Alternatively, patients achieving response may continue with treatment, those with progressive disease discontinue treatment and those with stable disease are randomised (Stadler 2007). The current design, incorporating randomisation of patients who are responding to treatment, may be more applicable to other disease areas where life-threatening consequences of discontinuing treatment may be less immediate, and there are fewer potential ethical implications associated with this.

4.7.2   Continuous outcome measure

No references identified.

4.7.3   Multinomial outcome measure

No references identified.

4.7.4   Time-to-event outcome measure

No references identified.

4.7.5   Ratio of times to progression

No references identified.

5

Treatment selection designs

Sarah Brown

The designs described within this chapter specifically address the question of treatment selection, that is, randomisation to multiple experimental treatment arms is incorporated. It is, however, also possible to consider treatment selection using single-arm or randomised phase II designs described in Chapters 3 and 4. In this respect the aim is to show that each experimental treatment has sufficient activity (and tolerability, if appropriate) before performing treatment selection. Treatment selection from those experimental arms found to be sufficiently active (and tolerable if appropriate) may then take place, for example, using selection designs such as those described by Sargent and Goldberg (2001) or Simon et al. (1985) (see Section 5.2.1 for further details). These designs select the most active treatment with a pre-specified probability of correct selection, according to the difference in activity observed between the experimental arms. Such an approach, combining these selection designs with other phase II designs, ensures that the treatments considered for selection have already passed pre-specified minimum activity criteria (and possibly tolerability criteria), prior to selection. Steinberg and Venzon provide an example of such an approach, as described in Section 5.2.2 (Steinberg and Venzon 2002). The efficiency of such an approach, as compared with the alternative treatment selection designs described within this chapter, should be considered in further detail on a trial-specific basis.

The designs within this chapter are organised as follows. First, designs including a control arm are described in Section 5.1, organised by design category and by outcome measure distribution. Second, in Section 5.2, designs that do not include a control arm are presented, again by design category and by outcome measure. Treatment selection designs that incorporate both activity *and* toxicity are presented separately in Section 6.4.

A Practical Guide to Designing Phase II Trials in Oncology, First Edition.
Sarah R. Brown, Walter M. Gregory, Chris Twelves and Julia Brown.
© 2014 John Wiley & Sons, Ltd. Published 2014 by John Wiley & Sons, Ltd.

5.1 Including a control arm

5.1.1 One-stage designs

5.1.1.1 Binary outcome measure

No references identified.

5.1.1.2 Continuous outcome measure

No references identified.

5.1.1.3 Multinomial outcome measure

Whitehead and Jaki (2009)

- One-stage, multinomial outcome, control arm
- Formal comparison with control for selection
- Programs noted as being available from authors
- No early termination

Whitehead and Jaki propose one- and two-stage designs for phase II trials based on ordered category outcomes, when the aim of the trial is to select a single treatment to take forward to phase III evaluation. The design is randomised to incorporate a formal comparison with a control arm, and hypothesis testing is based on the Mann–Whitney statistic. The treatment identified with the smallest p-value indicating a treatment effect is selected as the treatment to take forward for further investigation. Details of sample size and critical value calculation are provided, and R code is noted as being available from the authors to allow implementation. Specification of the worthwhile treatment effect and the small positive treatment effect that is not worth further investigation are required to be specified.

5.1.1.4 Time-to-event outcome measure

No references identified.

5.1.1.5 Ratio of times to progression

No references identified.

5.1.2 Two-stage designs

5.1.2.1 Binary outcome measure

Jung (2008)

- Two-stage, binary outcome, control arm
- Formal comparison with control for selection

- Programs noted as being available from author
- Early termination for lack of activity

Jung proposes a randomised controlled extension to Simon's optimal and minimax designs (Simon 1989), considering a binary outcome measure and incorporating early termination for lack of activity. The experimental arms are compared with the control arm at the end of stage 1 and treatments may be dropped for lack of activity. More than one experimental arm may therefore be taken forward to stage 2. If no treatments show improved activity over the control arm at the end of stage 1 the trial may be terminated for lack of activity. At the end of stage 2, all arms that pass the stage 2 cut-off boundaries compared to control are deemed worthy of further investigation. The selection design is an extension to the design described comparing a single experimental arm with a control. In the selection design the family-wise error rate, the probability of erroneously accepting an inactive treatment, is controlled. Programs to identify designs are available upon request from the author.

Jung and George (2009)

- Two-stage, binary outcome, control arm
- Formal comparison with control for selection
- Requires minimal programming
- Early termination for lack of activity

Jung and George propose methods of comparing treatment arms in a randomised phase II trial, where the intention is either to select one treatment from many for further evaluation or to determine whether a single treatment is worthy of evaluation compared to a control. The phase II design is based on a k-armed trial (with or without a control arm for selection) with each arm designed for independent evaluation following Simon's two-stage design (Simon 1989), or similar, based on historical control data, that is, no comparison is made with the control arm at this stage. Different designs (i.e. the same two-stage design but with different operating characteristics) may be used for different arms in the independent evaluation if deemed necessary. A treatment must be accepted via the independent evaluation before it can be considered for selection, at which point comparisons may be made with the control arm. p-Values are calculated to represent the probability that the difference between the arms being compared is at least some pre-defined minimal accepted difference, given the actual difference observed. The outcome measure used to select the better treatment is the same outcome measure used for evaluation of each arm independently, for example, tumour response. No software is detailed; however, detail is given which should allow implementation, and sufficient examples are also provided. The initial two-stage design can be calculated using software available for Simon's two-stage design.

5.1.2.2   Continuous outcome measure

Levy et al. (2006)

- Two-stage, continuous outcome, control arm
- No formal comparison with control for selection
- Requires programming
- No early termination; treatment selection at the end of stage 1

Levy et al. propose a randomised two-stage futility design incorporating treatment selection at the end of the first stage. At the end of the first stage the 'best' treatment is selected based on the treatment with the highest/lowest ('best') mean outcome, that is, no comparison with control is made here. Sample size for the first stage is calculated to give at least 80% probability of correct selection. Patients then continue to be randomised between control and the selected treatment, and data from the first stage is incorporated into the second-stage futility analysis, incorporating a bias correction. The null hypothesis is that the selected treatment reduces the mean response by at least x% compared to control; the alternative hypothesis is that the selected treatment reduces the mean response by less than x% compared to control (reflecting a futility design). Sample size and power calculation details are provided in appendices.

Shun et al. (2008)

- Two-stage, continuous outcome, control arm
- No formal comparison with control for treatment selection
- Requires programming
- No early termination at the end of stage 1

Shun et al. propose a phase II/III or two-stage treatment selection design where a single treatment is selected from two at the end of the first stage. Randomisation incorporates a control arm, with the intention of formal comparison at the end of the second stage only, that is, no formal comparison for treatment selection. Treatment selection is based on the experimental treatment with the highest/lowest ('best') mean outcome. A normal approximation approach is proposed to avoid complex numerical integration requirements. The design assumes that the treatment effects of the experimental treatments are *not* the same. The practical approach to timing of interim analysis addresses the need to perform this early in order to avoid type I error inflation and the need to perform this late enough such that there is a high probability of correctly selecting the better treatment. No software is noted as being available; however, detail is provided to allow implementation and a detailed example is given. The authors note that this design can be extended to binary and time-to-event outcome measures if the correlation between the final and interim test statistics is known.

5.1.2.3   Multinomial outcome measure

Sun et al. (2009)

- Two-stage, multinomial outcome, control arm

- Formal comparison with control

- Software noted as being available from author

- Early termination for lack of activity; early treatment selection

Sun and colleagues propose a randomised two-stage design based on Zee's single-arm multi-stage design with multinomial outcome measure (Zee et al. 1999), adjusting the rules such that a sufficiently high response rate *or* a sufficiently low early progressive disease rate should warrant further investigation of a treatment. Optimal and minimax designs are proposed following the methodology of Simon (1989), incorporating comparison with a control arm. Differences in response and progressive disease rates between control and experimental arms are compared. The authors note that the intention of the phase II trial is to screen for potential efficacy as opposed to identifying statistically significant differences compared with control. Patients are randomised between multiple experimental treatments and a control arm. At the end of the first stage only those treatments that pass the stopping boundaries for both response and progressive disease are continued to the second stage. If there is clear evidence that one treatment is better than the other, selection may take place at the end of the first stage. If, at the end of the second stage, there is no clear evidence that one experimental treatment is better than the other both arms may be considered for further evaluation. Detail is given regarding how to implement the designs in practice, and software is noted as being available by contacting the first author to allow identification of designs. The authors also note that the design may be extended to studies monitoring safety and efficacy simultaneously.

Whitehead and Jaki (2009)

- Two-stage, multinomial outcome, control arm

- Formal comparison with control for selection

- Programs noted as being available from authors

- No early termination

Whitehead and Jaki propose one- and two-stage designs for phase II trials based on ordered category outcomes, when the aim of the trial is to select a single treatment to take forward to phase III evaluation. The design is randomised to incorporate a formal comparison with a control arm, and hypothesis testing is based on the Mann–Whitney statistic. In the two-stage design, treatment selection takes place at the end of stage 1 whereby the treatment with the smallest p-value indicating a treatment effect is selected as the treatment to take forward to stage 2. In stage 2, patients are randomised between the selected treatment and control only. The final analysis at the end of stage

2 is based on all data available on patients in the control arm and the selected treatment arm. Details of sample size and critical value calculation are provided, and R code is noted as being available from the authors to allow implementation. Specification of the worthwhile treatment effect and the small positive treatment effect that is not worth further investigation are required to be specified.

5.1.2.4   Time-to-event outcome measure

No references identified.

5.1.2.5   Ratio of times to progression

No references identified.

5.1.3   Multi-stage designs

5.1.3.1   Binary outcome measure

No references identified.

5.1.3.2   Continuous outcome measure

Cheung (2009)

- Multi-stage, continuous outcome, control arm
- Formal comparison with control for treatment selection
- Requires programming
- Early treatment selection and early termination for lack of activity

Cheung describes an adaptive multi-arm, multi-stage selection design incorporating a control arm and considering a normally distributed outcome measure. Two multi-stage procedures are proposed: an extension of the sequential probability ratio test (SPRT) with a maximum sample size and a truncated sequential elimination procedure (ELIM). The SPRT method allows early selection of a treatment when there is evidence of increased activity compared to control, whereas the ELIM procedure also allows early termination of arms for lack of activity. The proposed procedures are compared with single-arm trials and the ELIM procedure is recommended over these, incorporating sample size reassessment at interim analyses. Cohort sizes between interim assessments may range from 1 to 10 with little impact on the design's operating characteristics. Sample size formulae are provided which will require implementing in order to identify the trial design.

5.1.3.3   Multinomial outcome measure

No references identified.

5.1.3.4   Time-to-event outcome measure

No references identified.

5.1.3.5   Ratio of times to progression

No references identified.

5.1.4   Continuous monitoring designs

No references identified.

5.1.5   Decision-theoretic designs

No references identified.

5.1.6   Three-outcome designs

No references identified.

5.1.7   Phase II/III designs – same primary outcome measure at phase II and phase III

The designs outlined within this section incorporate the same primary outcome measure for phase II assessment as that used for phase III. Although this may be seen as a seamless phase II/III approach, in effect it reflects a phase III trial with an early interim analysis on the primary outcome measure. In this setting, consideration should be given to the most appropriate outcome measure to use for both the phase II *and* phase III primary outcome. It is rare that efficacy in the phase III setting could be claimed on the basis of, for example, a binary outcome; rather, a time-to-event outcome is usually required in phase III trials.

5.1.7.1   Binary outcome measure

Bauer et al. (1998)

- Phase II/III, binary outcome, control arm

- Formal comparison with control for treatment selection

- Programs noted as being available from authors

- Early termination for efficacy at the end of phase II

Bauer and colleagues outline a simulation program for an adaptive two-stage design with application to phase II/III and dose finding. Two outcomes may be considered, with one primary variable on which formal hypothesis testing is performed and the other for which adaptations at the end of the first stage may be based on. The outcomes may be binary or continuous, or a combination. The same primary outcome measure is used at each analysis. Simulation is required to identify the best design according to various operating characteristics and the performance of different designs. A program is detailed (the focus of the manuscript) to allow implementation, which is noted as being available on request from the authors. At the end of the first stage the stage 1 hypothesis is tested, generating a p-value $p1$. At the end of the second stage the stage 2 hypothesis is tested using only data obtained from patients in stage 2, generating a p-value $p2$. The overall hypothesis is then tested combining $p1$ and $p2$ using Fisher's combination test (Fisher 1932). Application is given to phase II/III, with treatment selection at the end of stage 1: if the p-value is significant that at least one of the treatments is superior then the treatment with the 'best' outcome is considered in phase III. The trial may also terminate early for efficacy at the end of stage 1 if the p-value is significant at the stage 2 significance level.

Bauer and Kieser (1999)

- Phase II/III, binary outcome, control arm

- Formal comparison with control for treatment selection

- Programs noted as being available from author

- Early termination for efficacy at the end of phase II

Bauer and Kieser detail a design that incorporates formal comparison of each of the experimental arms with the control at the end of phase II (as well as testing whether *any* of the treatments are superior to control). The same primary outcome measure is used in both phases II and III. A fixed sample size is used for phase II, however the phase III sample size can be updated adaptively at the end of phase II. Stopping at the end of phase II is permissible for either lack of efficacy or early evidence of efficacy. The design also allows more than one treatment to be taken forward to phase III. At the end of phase II the sample size may be re-estimated and the test statistics to use at phase III are determined, according to the number of treatments taken forward and the hypotheses to be tested. The decision criterion at the end of phase III is based on Fisher's combination test (Fisher 1932) whereby the p-values from both phases are combined (as opposed to combining data from all patients). Simulation is required as detailed in Bauer et al. (1998), as above. Examples are given in the dose-finding setting and the authors note that the main advantage of this design is its flexibility and its control of the family-wise error rate. The design is similar to that detailed above (Bauer et al. 1998) with the exception that the current paper gives more detail relating to multiple comparisons between experimental treatments and control arm. When considering either of these two designs, it is advised that both papers be considered together since the software detailed in Bauer et al., above, is required to identify the design proposed here.

Stallard and Todd (2003)

- Phase II/III, binary outcome, control arm

- Formal comparison with control for treatment selection

- Programs noted as being available from authors
- Early termination for efficacy at the end of phase II

Stallard and Todd propose a design whereby patients from phase II are incorporated in the phase III analysis, and treatment selection at the end of phase II is based on the treatment with the largest test statistic using efficient scores and Fisher's information. A formal comparison is made between the selected treatment and control, and the trial may be terminated early for lack of efficacy or superiority at this stage. The type I error in the final phase III analysis is adjusted for the treatment selection in phase II. Overall sample size and phase II sample size are computed according to group-sequential phase III designs such as those described by Whitehead (1997). A computer program is noted as being available from the authors to calculate power for stopping boundaries, according to pre-specified group sizes. The authors note that the design is useful when one treatment is likely to be much better than the others at phase II, as opposed to taking multiple treatments to phase III. Consideration should also be given to the timing of the first interim analysis (i.e. phase II assessment). Too early and there is too little information, too late and there are too many patients enrolled and thus potentially wasted resources.

Kelly et al. (2005)

- Phase II/III, binary outcome, control arm
- Formal comparison with control for treatment selection
- Requires programming
- Early termination for efficacy and lack of efficacy during phase II

Kelly and colleagues propose an adaptation to the design proposed by Stallard and Todd (detailed above), such that more than one treatment may be selected at multiple stages within the phase II part of the trial. Treatments are evaluated for selection using Fisher's information and an efficient score statistic which may be applied to continuous, binary and failure time data. p-Values are calculated at each stage for comparison of the best treatment with control. Only treatments within a pre-specified margin of the efficient score statistic of the best treatment are continued to the next stage, and all other treatments are dropped. Patients are randomised between control and each of the treatments under investigation at each stage. The trial may stop for efficacy or lack of efficacy at each stage. The example given is based on the use of the triangular test described by Whitehead (1997), which uses expected Fisher's information to calculate operating characteristics.

Wang and Cui (2007)

- Phase II/III, binary outcome, control arm
- No formal comparison with control in phase II

- Requires programming
- No early termination during phase II

Wang and Cui outline a design whereby patients are randomised to each of the experimental treatments under investigation and a control arm, using response-adaptive randomisation (the paper is written in the context of dose selection but could be applied to treatment selection). The allocation ratios are calculated based on distance conditional powers (i.e. the probability that the event rate for the treatment under investigation is larger than some pre-specified fixed rate, based on the observed data and the fact that some patients will not yet have had their outcome observed). The treatment to which most patients have been randomised is deemed the most efficacious at the end of the recruitment period. This selected treatment is then formally compared with the control treatment, forming the phase III comparison. This design uses binary outcome measures such as treatment response, for both the phase II treatment selection and the phase III formal comparison; although it is noted that continuous outcomes may be used. Simulation is required to investigate the design parameters, with sample size calculated based on the phase III comparison. The design may be implemented with the development of programs based on formulae provided.

5.1.7.2   Continuous outcome measure

Bretz et al. (2006)

- Phase II/III, continuous outcome, control arm
- Formal comparison with control for treatment selection
- Minimal programming required
- Early termination for efficacy or lack of efficacy at the end of phase II

Bretz and colleagues outline a phase II/III design which allows treatment selection at the interim assessment (i.e. at the end of phase II). The design allows data from the first stage to be incorporated into the final analysis. Formal comparisons between control and experimental treatments are performed at the end of each stage. Early termination is permitted at the end of the first stage (i.e. at the end of phase II) for lack of efficacy or for early evidence of efficacy. Also at this time, if the study is to be continued to phase III, adaptations to the design of the trial may be made such as sample size reassessment based on the data observed to date. Final analysis includes data from both stages, with decision criteria based on a combination of test results (i.e. using methods such as Fisher's product test of the conditional error function). The closure principle is incorporated, such that a hypothesis is only rejected if it and all associated intersection hypotheses are also rejected. Sample size formulae are given to allow calculation. The design may be extended to multiple stages, in which case early termination during the phase II aspect may be incorporated.

Bauer et al. (1998)

- Phase II/III, continuous outcome, control arm

- Formal comparison with control for treatment selection

- Programs noted as being available from authors

- Early termination for efficacy at the end of phase II

Bauer and colleagues outline a simulation program for an adaptive two-stage design with application to phase II/III and dose finding. Two outcomes may be considered, with one primary variable on which formal hypothesis testing is performed and the other for which adaptations at the end of the first stage may be based on. The outcomes may be binary or continuous, or a combination. The same primary outcome measure is used at each analysis. Simulation is required to identify the best design according to various operating characteristics and the performance of different designs. A program is detailed (the focus of the manuscript) to allow implementation, which is noted as being available on request from the authors. At the end of the first stage the stage 1 hypothesis is tested, generating a p-value $p1$. At the end of the second stage the stage 2 hypothesis is tested using only data obtained from patients in stage 2, generating a p-value $p2$. The overall hypothesis is then tested combining $p1$ and $p2$ using Fisher's combination test (Fisher 1932). Application is given to phase II/III, with treatment selection at the end of stage 1: if the p-value is significant that at least one of the treatments is superior then the treatment with the 'best' outcome is considered in phase III. The trial may also terminate early for efficacy at the end of stage 1 if the p-value is significant at the stage 2 significance level.

Bauer and Kieser (1999)

- Phase II/III, continuous outcome, control arm

- Formal comparison with control for treatment selection

- Programs noted as being available from author

- Early termination for efficacy at the end of phase II

Bauer and Kieser detail a design that incorporates formal comparison of each of the experimental arms with the control at the end of phase II (as well as testing whether *any* of the treatments are superior to control). The same primary outcome measure is used in both phases II and III. A fixed sample size is used for phase II, however the phase III sample size can be updated adaptively at the end of phase II. Stopping at the end of phase II is permissible for either lack of efficacy or early evidence of efficacy and is based on p-value calculation. The design also allows more than one treatment to be taken forward to phase III. At the end of phase II the sample size may be re-estimated and the test statistics to use at phase III are determined, according to the number of treatments taken forward and the hypotheses to be tested. The decision criterion at the end of phase III is based on Fisher's combination test

(Fisher 1932) whereby the *p*-values from both phases are combined (as opposed to combining data from all patients). Simulation is required as detailed in Bauer et al. (1998), as above. Examples are given in the dose-finding setting and the authors note that the main advantage of this design is its flexibility and its control of the family-wise error rate. The design is similar to that detailed above (Bauer et al. 1998) with the exception that the current paper gives more detail relating to the multiple comparisons between experimental treatments and control arm. When considering either of these two designs, it is advised that both papers be considered together since the software detailed in Bauer et al., above, is required to identify the design proposed here.

Stallard and Todd (2003)

- Phase II/III, continuous outcome, control arm

- Formal comparison with control for treatment selection

- Programs noted as being available from authors

- Early termination for efficacy at the end of phase II

Stallard and Todd propose a design whereby patients from phase II are incorporated in the phase III analysis, and treatment selection at the end of phase II is based on the treatment with the largest test statistic using efficient scores and Fisher's information. A formal comparison is made between the selected treatment and control, and the trial may be terminated early for lack of efficacy or superiority at this stage. The type I error in the final phase III analysis is adjusted for the treatment selection in phase II. Overall sample size and phase II sample size are computed according to group-sequential phase III designs such as those described by Whitehead (1997). A computer program is noted as being available from the authors to calculate power for stopping boundaries, according to pre-specified group sizes. The authors note that the design is useful when one treatment is likely to be much better than the others at phase II, as opposed to taking multiple treatments to phase III. Consideration should also be given to the timing of the first interim analysis (i.e. phase II assessment). Too early and there is too little information, too late and there are too many patients enrolled and thus potentially wasted resources.

Kelly et al. (2005)

- Phase II/III, continuous outcome, control arm

- Formal comparison with control for treatment selection

- Requires programming

- Early termination for efficacy and lack of efficacy during phase II

Kelly and colleagues propose an adaptation to the design proposed by Stallard and Todd (detailed above), such that more than one treatment may be selected at multiple stages within the phase II part of the trial. Treatments are evaluated for selection using Fisher's information and an efficient score statistic which may be applied to continuous, binary and failure time data. p-Values are calculated at each stage for comparison of the best treatment with control. Only treatments within a pre-specified margin of the efficient score statistic of the best treatment are continued to the next stage, and all other treatments are dropped. Patients are randomised between control and each of the treatments under investigation at each stage. The trial may stop for efficacy or lack of efficacy at each stage. The example given is based on the use of the triangular test described by Whitehead (1997), which uses expected Fisher's information to calculate operating characteristics.

Wang (2006)

- Phase II/III, continuous outcome, control arm

- Formal comparison with control for treatment selection

- Requires programming

- Early termination for efficacy at the end of phase II

Wang proposes an adaptive design with treatment selection at the end of phase II. Patients are randomised between control and each of the experimental treatments under investigation in phase II. The design controls the overall type I error and allows the conditional error function of the phase III trial to depend on the data observed during phase II. Maximum sample sizes are required to be specified and simulations performed to evaluate expected sample size. The identification of the optimal design requires detailed numerical integration. At the end of the first stage the treatment with the largest test statistic is selected to take forward to phase III; however, the trial could also be stopped at this point (i.e. at the end of phase II) for efficacy or lack of efficacy. There is formal comparison between each of the experimental arms and the control arm at the end of phase II, and as long as at least one experimental treatment has sufficient activity, a treatment is selected for further testing in phase III (or selected as being superior if significant enough). The design has been implemented in R and formulae are given to allow this to be implemented in other software, therefore the design would need programming.

Wang and Cui (2007)

- Phase II/III, continuous outcome, control arm

- No formal comparison with control in phase II

- Requires programming

- No early termination during phase II

Wang and Cui outline a design whereby patients are randomised to each of the experimental treatments under investigation and a control arm, using response-adaptive randomisation (the paper is written in the context of dose selection but could be applied to treatment selection). The allocation ratios are calculated based on distance conditional powers (i.e. the probability that the treatment effect for the treatment under investigation is larger than some pre-specified fixed value, based on the observed data and the fact that some patients will not yet have had their outcome observed). The treatment to which most patients have been randomised is deemed the most efficacious at the end of the recruitment period. This selected treatment is then formally compared with the control treatment, forming the phase III comparison. This design as detailed uses binary outcome measures such as treatment response, for both the phase II treatment selection and the phase III formal comparison, although it is noted that continuous outcomes may be used. Simulation is required to investigate the design parameters, with sample size calculated based on the phase III comparison. The design may be implemented with the development of programs based on formulae provided.

Shun et al. (2008)

- Phase II/III, continuous outcome, control arm

- No formal comparison with control for treatment selection

- Requires programming

- No early termination at the end of phase II

Shun et al. propose a phase II/III or two-stage treatment selection design where a single treatment is selected from two at the end of the first stage. Randomisation incorporates a control arm, with the intention of formal comparison at the end of the second stage only, that is, no formal comparison for treatment selection. Treatment selection is based on the experimental treatment with the highest/lowest ('best') mean outcome. A normal approximation approach is proposed to avoid complex numerical integration requirements. The design assumes that the treatment effects of the experimental treatments are *not* the same. The practical approach to timing of interim analysis addresses the need to perform this early in order to avoid type I error inflation, and the need to perform this late enough such that there is a high probability of correctly selecting the better treatment. No software is noted as being available; however, detail is provided to allow implementation and a detailed example is given. The authors note that this design can be extended to binary and time-to-event outcome measures if the correlation between the final and interim test statistics is known.

5.1.7.3 Multinomial outcome measure

Whitehead and Jaki (2009)

- Phase II/III, multinomial outcome, control arm

- Formal comparison with control for selection

- Programs noted as being available from authors

- No early termination during phase II

Whitehead and Jaki propose one- and two-stage designs for phase II trials based on ordered category outcomes, when the aim of the trial is to select a single treatment to take forward to phase III evaluation. The authors note that the two-stage design detailed may be applied to the phase II/III setting, although refinements to the design may be required including the use of different outcome measures for treatment selection and final analysis. The design is randomised to incorporate a formal comparison with a control arm, and hypothesis testing is based on the Mann–Whitney statistic. In the phase II/III setting, treatment selection takes place at the end of stage 1, that is, phase II, whereby the treatment with the smallest p-value indicating a treatment effect is selected as the treatment to take forward to stage 2, that is, phase III. Early termination for lack of activity is permitted at the end of phase II. During phase III, patients are randomised between the selected treatment and control only. The final analysis at the end of phase III is based on all data available on patients in the control arm and the selected treatment arm. Details of sample size and critical value calculation are provided, and R code is noted as being available from the authors to allow implementation. Specification of the worthwhile treatment effect and the small positive treatment effect that is not worth further investigation are required to be specified.

5.1.7.4   Time-to-event outcome measure

Bauer and Kieser (1999)

- Phase II/III, time-to-event outcome, control arm

- Formal comparison with control for treatment selection

- Programs noted as being available from author

- Early termination for efficacy at the end of phase II

Bauer and Kieser detail a design that incorporates formal comparison of each of the experimental arms with the control at the end of phase II (as well as testing whether *any* of the treatments are superior to control). The same primary outcome measure is used in both phases II and III. A fixed sample size is used for phase II, however the phase III sample size can be updated adaptively at the end of phase II. Stopping at the end of phase II is permissible for either lack of efficacy or early evidence of efficacy and is based on p-value calculation. The design also allows more than one treatment to be taken forward to phase III. At the end of phase II the sample size may be re-estimated and the test statistics to use at phase III are determined, according to the number of treatments taken forward and the hypotheses to be tested. The decision criterion at the end of phase III is based on Fisher's combination test (Fisher 1932) whereby the p-values from both phases are combined (as opposed to combining data from all patients). Simulation is required as detailed in Bauer et al. (1998). Examples are given in the dose-finding setting and the authors note that the main advantage of this design is its flexibility and its control of the family-wise error rate. When considering this design, it is advised that the detail provided by Bauer et al.

(1998) also be reviewed since this paper outlines the software required to identify the design proposed here.

Stallard and Todd (2003)

- Phase II/III, time-to-event outcome, control arm
- Formal comparison with control for treatment selection
- Programs noted as being available from authors
- Early termination for efficacy at the end of phase II

Stallard and Todd propose a design whereby patients from phase II are incorporated in the phase III analysis, and treatment selection at the end of phase II is based on the treatment with the largest test statistic using efficient scores and Fisher's information. A formal comparison is made between the selected treatment and control, and the trial may be terminated early for lack of efficacy or superiority at this stage. The type I error in the final phase III analysis is adjusted for the treatment selection in phase II. Overall sample size and phase II sample size are computed according to group-sequential phase III designs such as those described by Whitehead (1997). A computer program is noted as being available from the authors to calculate power for stopping boundaries, according to pre-specified group sizes. The authors note that the design is useful when one treatment is likely to be much better than the others at phase II, as opposed to taking multiple treatments to phase III. Consideration should also be given to the timing of the first interim analysis (i.e. phase II assessment). Too early and there is too little information, too late and there are too many patients enrolled and thus potentially wasted resources.

Kelly et al. (2005)

- Phase II/III, time-to-event outcome, control arm
- Formal comparison with control for treatment selection
- Requires programming
- Early termination for efficacy and lack of efficacy during phase II

Kelly and colleagues propose an adaptation to the design proposed by Stallard and Todd (detailed above), such that more than one treatment may be selected at multiple stages within the phase II part of the trial. Treatments are evaluated for selection using Fisher's information and an efficient score statistic which may be applied to continuous, binary and failure time data. p-Values are calculated at each stage for comparison of the best treatment with control. Only treatments within a pre-specified margin of the efficient score statistic of the best treatment are continued to the next stage, and all other treatments are dropped. Patients are randomised between control and each of the treatments under investigation at each stage. The trial may stop for efficacy or lack of efficacy at each stage. The example given is based on the use of the triangular test described by Whitehead (1997), which uses expected Fisher's information to calculate operating characteristics.

5.1.7.5   Ratio of times to progression

No references identified.

5.1.8   Phase II/III designs – different primary outcome measures at phase II and phase III

The literature described within this section considers designs whereby different primary outcome measures are used for phase II and for phase III. Here the phase II primary outcome measure should be selected based on the discussions provided in Chapter 2, as this is not intended to be used for phase III decision-making.

5.1.8.1   Binary outcome measure

Todd and Stallard (2005)

- Phase II/III, binary outcome, control arm

- Formal comparison with control for treatment selection

- Programs noted as being available from the authors

- No early termination during phase II

Todd and Stallard describe a design where treatment selection occurs at the first interim assessment (phase II) based on comparison of a short-term outcome measure for each of the treatments versus control. Patients are randomised to each of the experimental treatments and control during phase II, and then to the selected treatment and the control during phase III. Phase III is carried out in a group-sequential manner, with the experimental treatment compared to control in terms of a longer term outcome measure. Selection at phase II is based on the treatment with the largest test statistic, that is, there is formal comparison with control but the study may only be terminated for lack of activity at this stage. The trial protocol remains the same throughout the study; therefore, patients in phase II can be incorporated in phase III. Required treatment effects (clinically significant), treatment effects that are still desirable but not clinically significant and expected correlation between phase II and III outcome measures are all required to identify the complete phase II/III design. Formulae are given and programs are noted as being available from the authors to calculate stopping boundaries.

5.1.8.2   Continuous outcome measure

Todd and Stallard (2005)

- Phase II/III, continuous outcome, control arm

- Formal comparison with control for treatment selection

- Programs noted as being available from authors

- No early termination during phase II

Todd and Stallard describe a design where treatment selection occurs at the first interim assessment (phase II) based on comparison of a short-term outcome measure for each of the treatments versus control. Patients are randomised to each of the experimental treatments and control during phase II, and then to the selected treatment and the control during phase III. Phase III is carried out in a group-sequential manner, with the experimental treatment compared to control in terms of a longer term outcome measure. Selection at phase II is based on the treatment with the largest test statistic, that is, there is formal comparison with control but the study may only be terminated for lack of activity at this stage. The trial protocol remains the same throughout the study; therefore, patients in phase II can be incorporated in phase III. Required treatment effects (clinically significant), treatment effects that are still desirable but not clinically significant and expected correlation between phase II and III outcome measures are all required to identify the complete phase II/III design. Formulae are given and programs are noted as being available from the authors to calculate stopping boundaries.

Liu and Pledger (2005)

- Phase II/III, continuous outcome, control arm

- Formal comparison with control for treatment selection

- Requires programming

- No early termination during phase II

Liu and Pledger detail a phase II/III design in the dose-finding context where patients are randomised to different doses and a placebo–control with the intention of dose selection, as well as an adaptive two-stage phase II/III design where the intention of phase II is to determine whether or not to continue to phase III, for a single experimental treatment. Short-term continuous outcome measures are used at the end of phase II to 'prune' the doses and to perform sample size adjustment for the second stage (phase III), and long-term continuous outcome measures are used to estimate the dose–response curve to calculate trend statistics for the analysis of the phase III (and also at the end of phase II). Patients continue to be randomised to all doses for a short period of phase III during the first analysis for dose selection at the end of phase II (i.e. there is no break in recruitment for phase II analysis), at which point more than one dose may be carried forward. The treatment effect required to be observed is the same for both short- and long-term outcome measures and needs to be pre-specified, along with prior information on probability of success for each dose, standard deviation for each outcome measure, the time period between enrolment of the first patient and the first analysis and the likely recruitment in this period. This information is used to generate the operating characteristics of the design. Formulae are given which would need to be implemented in order to identify the design. The design offers flexibility in that the second stage (phase III) sample size may be calculated based on updated data from the first stage (phase II), and adaptation rules do not need to be specified in advance.

Shun et al. (2008)

- Phase II/III, continuous outcome, control arm

- No formal comparison with control for treatment selection

- Requires programming

- No early termination at the end of phase II

Shun et al. propose a phase II/III or two-stage treatment selection design where a single treatment is selected from two at the end of the first stage (i.e. phase II). Randomisation incorporates a control arm, with the intention of formal comparison at the end of the second stage only, that is, no formal comparison for treatment selection. Treatment selection is based on the experimental treatment with the highest/lowest ('best') mean outcome. A normal approximation approach is proposed to avoid complex numerical integration requirements. Where a different outcome measure is used during phase II for treatment selection, the correlation between the phase II and III outcome measures must be specified. The design assumes that the treatment effects of the experimental treatments are *not* the same. The practical approach to timing of interim analysis addresses the need to perform this early in order to avoid type I error inflation, and the need to perform this late enough such that there is a high probability of correctly selecting the better treatment. No software is noted as being available; however, detail is provided to allow implementation and a detailed example is given. The authors note that this design can be extended to binary and time-to-event outcome measures if the correlation between the final and interim test statistics is known.

5.1.8.3   Multinomial outcome measure

No references identified.

5.1.8.4   Time-to-event outcome measure

Royston et al. (2003)

- Phase II/III, time-to-event outcome, control arm

- Formal comparison with control for treatment selection

- Some programming required before using standard software

- No early termination during phase II

Royston and colleagues outline a multi-arm, two-stage design aimed at identifying treatments worthy of further consideration at the end of the first stage by comparing each treatment with a control arm using an intermediate outcome measure of treatment activity. Only those treatments showing sufficient improvement in activity over control are continued to the second stage, at the end of which the treatments are each compared with control using an outcome measure of primary interest (i.e. different to that used at the end of the first stage). Data from both stages of the trial are incorporated in the final analysis at the end of stage 2. The design may be seen to reflect a seamless phase II/III design with treatment selection at the end of phase II, allowing more than one treatment to be continued into phase III. In evaluating the operating characteristics of the design, an estimate of the correlation between the treatment effects on the intermediate and final outcome measures is required. The authors propose an empirical approach to identifying this correlation using bootstrap resampling of previous data sets, thus the design requires data of this type to be available in order to allow implementation.

Todd and Stallard (2005)

- Phase II/III, time-to-event outcome, control arm

- Formal comparison with control for treatment selection

- Programs noted as being available from authors

- No early termination during phase II

Todd and Stallard describe a design where treatment selection occurs at the first interim assessment (phase II) based on comparison of a short-term outcome measure for each of the treatments versus control. Patients are randomised to each of the experimental treatments and control during phase II, and then to the selected treatment and the control during phase III. Phase III is carried out in a group-sequential manner, with the experimental treatment compared to control in terms of a longer term outcome measure. Selection at phase II is based on the treatment with the largest test statistic, that is, there is formal comparison with control but the study may only be terminated for lack of activity at this stage. The trial protocol remains the same throughout the study therefore patients in phase II can be incorporated in phase III. Required treatment effects (clinically significant), treatment effects that are still desirable but not clinically significant and expected correlation between phase II and III outcome measures are all required to identify the complete phase II/III design. Formulae are given and programs are noted as being available from the authors to calculate stopping boundaries.

5.1.8.5   Ratio of times to progression

No references identified.

5.1.9   Randomised discontinuation designs

No references identified.

5.2 Not including a control arm

5.2.1 One-stage designs

5.2.1.1 Binary outcome measure

Whitehead (1985)

- One-stage, binary outcome, no control arm

- Requires programming

- No early termination

Whitehead discusses a phase II selection design when there are a number of treatments available for study, currently and expected in the near future, and a fixed number of patients available over a period of time. Patients are randomised to the treatments currently available and new treatments may be entered as they become available. A given number of patients are recruited to each treatment and analysis takes place when all treatments have been considered. The design, for which no software is detailed but for which formulae are given to allow implementation, identifies the optimal number of treatments (t) and patients per treatment (n) such that nt = total number of patients available. The examples given consider trials including around 10 treatments, 6 patients per treatment, that is, 60 patients in total. Analysis takes the form of an appropriate statistical model, fitting treatment as a covariate and incorporating other prognostic variables as necessary. The treatment with the largest estimated beneficial effect is then selected for further investigation in phase III. The design allows modification such that more than one treatment may be taken forward and such that cut-off boundaries may be incorporated to ensure a pre-specified level of success. Any outcome measure distribution may be considered. No control patients are incorporated and no assessment of risk of a false-negative result is considered. It is noted that when only a few treatments are to be tested and when the number of patients available is plentiful, this design may be less appropriate.

Simon et al. (1985)

- One-stage, binary outcome, no control arm

- Software available

- No early termination

Simon et al. detail a selection procedure based on correctly selecting the treatment with the higher event rate when the difference in event rates is at least d, some pre-specified amount. The design proposed will always select a treatment, even if the differences are $<d$, but will do so with less assurance that the correct treatment is being selected. The design does not include a pre-specified minimum level of activity; however, it may be applied as an addition to another trial design establishing minimum levels of activity prior to treatment selection (as described in the introduction to this

chapter). The design is easily implemented in statistical programming software such as SAS and is available in Machin et al (2008).

Sargent and Goldberg (2001)

- One-stage, binary outcome, no control arm
- Requires programming
- No early termination

Sargent and Goldberg propose a similar treatment selection design to Simon et al., described above. The treatment with the higher event rate is selected when the difference between treatments in the event rate is at least d (required to be pre-specified). If the difference is less than d, other criteria for selection can be used. Sample size is selected by considering the probability that the better treatment is correctly selected. Treatments do not have to pass given boundaries for minimum activity, it is simply necessary for one treatment to be better than the other by at least d. Sample size can be reduced by incorporating allowance to correctly pick the better treatment when the result is ambiguous, that is, when the difference between treatments is less than d, assume that, for example, 50% of the time the better treatment would correctly be chosen based on other criteria. As described for the design proposed by Simon et al., this design does not need to operate alone and can be used in conjunction with other trial designs to ensure minimum levels of activity and to generate sample size. The design is easily implemented in statistical programming software such as SAS.

5.2.1.2   Continuous outcome measure

Whitehead (1985)

- One-stage, continuous outcome, no control arm
- Requires programming
- No early termination

Whitehead discusses a phase II selection design when there are a number of treatments available for study, currently and expected in the near future, and a fixed number of patients available over a period of time. Patients are randomised to the treatments currently available and new treatments may be entered as they become available. A given number of patients are recruited to each treatment and analysis takes place when all treatments have been considered. The design, for which no software is detailed but for which formulae are given to allow implementation, identifies the optimal number of treatments (t) and patients per treatment (n) such that $nt = $ total number of patients available. The examples given consider trials including around 10 treatments, 6 patients per treatment, that is, 60 patients in total. Analysis takes the form of an appropriate statistical model, fitting treatment as a covariate and incorporating other prognostic variables as necessary. The treatment with the largest estimated beneficial effect is then selected for further investigation in phase III. The design allows modification such that more than one treatment may be taken forward and such that cut-off boundaries may be incorporated to ensure a pre-specified level of success. Any outcome measure distribution may be considered. No control patients are incorporated and no assessment of risk of a false-negative result is considered. It is noted that when only a few treatments are to be tested and when the number of patients available is plentiful, this design may be less appropriate.

5.2.1.3   Multinomial outcome measure

No references identified.

5.2.1.4   Time-to-event outcome measure

Whitehead (1985)

- One-stage, time-to-event outcome, no control arm

- Requires programming

- No early termination

Whitehead discusses a phase II selection design when there are a number of treatments available for study, currently and expected in the near future, and a fixed number of patients available over a period of time. Patients are randomised to the treatments currently available and new treatments may be entered as they become available. A given number of patients are recruited to each treatment and analysis takes place when all treatments have been considered. The design, for which no software is detailed but for which formulae are given to allow implementation, identifies the optimal number of treatments (t) and patients per treatment (n) such that $nt =$ total number of patients available. The examples given consider trials including around 10 treatments, 6 patients per treatment, that is, 60 patients in total. Analysis takes the form of an appropriate statistical model, fitting treatment as a covariate and incorporating other prognostic variables as necessary. The treatment with the largest estimated beneficial effect is then selected for further investigation in phase III. The design allows modification such that more than one treatment may be taken forward and such that cut-off boundaries may be incorporated to ensure a pre-specified level of success. Any outcome measure distribution may be considered. No control patients are incorporated and no assessment of risk of a false-negative result is considered. It is noted that when only a few treatments are to be tested and when the number of patients available is plentiful, this design may be less appropriate.

5.2.1.5   Ratio of times to progression

No references identified.

5.2.2   Two-stage designs

5.2.2.1   Binary outcome measure

Weiss and Hokanson (1984)

- Two-stage, binary outcome, no control arm

- Standard software available

- Early termination for lack of activity

Weiss and Hokanson discuss the concept of integrated phase II trials to minimise the enrolment of an excessive number of patients into trials of potentially ineffective drugs. It is assumed that a number of treatments are available for investigation at the same time, which are ranked to determine which treatment should be assessed first in a sequence of integrated trials. The first cohort of n_1 patients are recruited to treatment 1 and followed up for response, during which the next cohort of n_1 patients are recruited to treatment 2, and so on. If a pre-specified number of responses are observed in any of the treatment arms from the first n_1 patients in that cohort, recruitment to further treatment arms is halted and a further n_2 patients are recruited to the treatment on which the responses were observed, essentially following an integrated scheme of multiple trials based on Gehan's design (Gehan 1961). The aim of the process is to assess each treatment individually for its inclusion in a phase III trial, as opposed to selecting one of the treatments alone to investigate further. As such, at the end of the integrated process, a number of treatments may be deemed worthy of further investigation.

Steinberg and Venzon (2002)

- Two-stage, binary outcome, no control arm

- Requires programming if design not in tables

- Early treatment selection permitted

Steinberg and Venzon propose an early selection design which may be used in conjunction with a single-arm phase II trial design (to generate sample size; the authors use Simon's two-stage design as an example). The proposed design incorporates assessment of two experimental treatments at the end of stage 1, selecting the superior treatment as the treatment with an event rate at least $x\%$ higher than the other treatment, with probability of correct selection z (x and z require pre-specifying). Tables are given to identify the required difference in number of events observed between the two arms to select the superior treatment early. If no treatment is selected at the end of stage 1, the trial continues to randomise between the two treatments with selection at the end, otherwise if a treatment is selected, the trial continues recruiting patients to that arm to the desired number of patients under the underlying design. When used in combination with, for example,

Simon's two-stage design, each treatment arm must independently pass the stopping boundaries at each stage to be evaluable for selection. This design may be considered over single-stage selection designs to enable treatment selection as early as possible.

Logan (2005)

- Two-stage, binary outcome, no control arm
- Requires programming if design not in tables
- Early termination for lack of activity

Logan proposes a two-stage selection design based on an adaptation of Simon's two-stage design (Simon 1989), as applied to a randomised selection trial. Treatments that do not pass the stopping criteria at the end of the first stage are dropped, and the sample size for the second stage is adapted based on the number of treatments remaining for stage 2, up to a maximum sample size. Since the second-stage sample size is adaptive, the cut-off boundaries for the second stage are also dependent on the number of treatments continuing. The intention is that at the end of the second stage, additional selection criteria may be applied to those treatments successfully passing the final stopping criteria, in the case of more than one treatment. The proposed design offers a saving in the total number of patients as compared to Simon's designs, when it is anticipated that not all treatments will be highly active. Tables of sample sizes and stopping boundaries are presented for various scenarios; however, additional designs require computing.

Jung and George (2009)

- Two-stage, binary outcome, no control arm
- Requires minimal programming
- Early termination for lack of activity

Jung and George propose methods of comparing treatment arms in a randomised phase II trial, where the intention is either to select one treatment from many for further evaluation or to determine whether a single treatment is worthy of evaluation compared to a control. The phase II design is based on a k-armed trial (with or without a control arm for selection) with each arm designed for independent evaluation following Simon's two-stage design (Simon 1989), or similar, based on historical control data. Different designs (i.e. the same two-stage design but with different operating characteristics) may be used for different arms in the independent evaluation if deemed necessary. A treatment must be accepted via the independent evaluation before it can be considered for selection, at which point between-arm comparisons are made. p-Values are calculated to represent the probability that the difference between the arms being compared is at least some pre-defined minimal accepted difference, given the actual difference observed. The outcome measure used to select the better treatment is the same outcome measure used for evaluation of each arm independently, for example, tumour response. No software is detailed; however, detail is given which should allow implementation, and sufficient examples are also provided. The initial two-stage design can be calculated using software available for Simon's two-stage design.

5.2.2.2   Continuous outcome measure

No references identified.

5.2.2.3   Multinomial outcome measure

No references identified.

5.2.2.4   Time-to-event outcome measure

No references identified.

5.2.2.5   Ratio of times to progression

No references identified.

5.2.3   Multi-stage designs

5.2.3.1   Binary outcome measure

Thall et al. (2000)

- Multi-stage, binary outcome, no control arm

- Requires programming (simulation programs noted as being available from author)

- No early termination (multi-stage randomisation)

Thall et al. outline a design for treatment *strategy* selection that incorporates response-adaptive randomisation within each patient, that is, future treatment strategies for each patient depend on the treatments they have already received, and their responses. This design is multi-stage in nature since patients are randomised at various stages throughout their treatment schedule. Sample size requires investigation via simulation, and the authors note that sample size should be determined empirically rather than using simpler methods. Response is categorised as success or failure, the criteria for which can be different for different stages of treatment. The 'best' treatment strategy is selected as that with the largest estimated success probability, which can be assessed by considering responses to multiple treatment strategies for each patient.

5.2.3.2   Continuous outcome measure

No references identified.

5.2.3.3   Multinomial outcome measure

No references identified.

5.2.3.4   Time-to-event outcome measure

Cheung and Thall (2002)

- Multi-stage, time-to-event outcome, no control arm

- Programs noted as being available from authors

- Early termination for activity or lack of activity

Cheung and Thall propose a Bayesian sequential-adaptive procedure for continuous monitoring, which may be extended to assessment after cohorts of more than 1 patient, that is, multi-stage. The outcome measure of interest is a binary indicator of a composite time-to-event outcome, utilising all the censored and uncensored observations at each interim assessment. Continuous monitoring based on the approximate posterior (CMAP) is used following Thall and Simon (1994b). The design can incorporate multiple competing and non-competing outcomes. Early termination of each treatment is permitted for activity or lack of activity; however, a treatment may also be dropped if it is inferior to the other treatments. Selection is based on the treatment with the largest success probability. R programs are noted as being available from the authors to allow implementation of the design. This design enables data to be incorporated on all patients at each interim assessment without all follow-up data being obtained and may therefore be used when follow-up of each patient is for a non-trivial period of time.

5.2.3.5   Ratio of times to progression

No references identified.

5.2.4   Continuous monitoring designs

5.2.4.1   Binary outcome measure

No references identified.

5.2.4.2   Continuous outcome measure

No references identified.

5.2.4.3   Multinomial outcome measure

No references identified.

5.2.4.4   Time-to-event outcome measure

Cheung and Thall (2002)

- Continuous monitoring, time-to-event outcome
- Programs noted as being available from authors
- Early termination for activity or lack of activity

Cheung and Thall propose a Bayesian sequential-adaptive procedure for continuous monitoring, which may be extended to assessment after cohorts of more than 1 patient, that is, multi-stage. The outcome measure of interest is a binary indicator of a composite time-to-event outcome, utilising all the censored and uncensored observations at each interim assessment. Continuous monitoring based on the approximate posterior (CMAP) is used following Thall and Simon (1994b). The design can incorporate multiple competing and non-competing outcomes. Early termination of each treatment is permitted for activity or lack of activity; however, a treatment may also be dropped if it is inferior to the other treatments. Selection is based on the treatment with the largest success probability. R programs are noted as being available from the authors to allow implementation of the design. This design enables data to be incorporated on all patients at each interim assessment without all follow-up data being obtained, and may therefore be used when follow-up of each patient is for a non-trivial period of time.

5.2.4.5   Ratio of times to progression

No references identified.

5.2.5   Decision-theoretic designs

No references identified.

5.2.6   Three-outcome designs

No references identified.

5.2.7   Phase II/III designs – same primary outcome measure at phase II and phase III

As described in Section 5.1.7, the designs outlined within this section incorporate the same primary outcome measure for phase II assessment as that used for phase III. Although this may be seen as seamless phase II/III approach, in effect it reflects a phase III trial with an early interim analysis on the primary outcome measure. In this setting, consideration should be given to the most appropriate outcome measure to use for both the phase II *and* phase III primary outcomes. It is rare that efficacy in the phase III setting could be claimed on the basis of, for example, a binary outcome; rather, a time-to-event outcome is usually required in phase III trials.

5.2.7.1 Binary outcome measure

Whitehead (1986)

- Phase II/III, binary outcome, no control arm in phase II

- Program available

- No early termination during phase II

Whitehead proposes a phase II/III selection design with a binary outcome at both phases. Randomisation in phase II is between experimental treatments only, and the treatment with the largest event rate is selected as the treatment to be taken forward to phase III, where randomisation then occurs between the selected treatment and a control. The selection of a treatment for phase III does not incorporate stopping boundaries for minimum levels of activity. Sample size is based on maximum available and is justified in terms of the probability of observing a significant result at phase III. A FORTRAN program is written to determine the optimal split of patients between phases II and III, and formulae are also provided in the appendices of the manuscript to detail this.

5.2.7.2 Continuous outcome measure

No references identified.

5.2.7.3 Multinomial outcome measure

No references identified.

5.2.7.4 Time-to-event outcome measure

No references identified.

5.2.7.5 Ratio of times to progression

No references identified.

5.2.8 Randomised discontinuation designs

No references identified.

6

Designs incorporating toxicity as a primary outcome

Sarah Brown

This chapter outlines the phase II designs available for trials where the primary outcome of interest is a joint outcome of both activity and toxicity or where toxicity is assessed alone. Section 6.1 outlines designs that incorporate a control arm, and Section 6.2 outlines those designs with no control arm, both organised by design category and by outcome measure distribution for the activity endpoint. Also, as discussed in Chapter 2, designs are available that address the option of using toxicity alone as the primary outcome measure in a phase II trial. These designs are described in Section 6.3 and may be considered as an add-on to a trial designed to assess activity. Finally, designs that incorporate both activity and toxicity for the purpose of treatment selection, that is, where there are multiple experimental treatments, are presented in Section 6.4.

6.1   Including a control arm

6.1.1   One-stage designs

6.1.1.1   Binary outcome measure

Thall and Cheng (1999)

- One-stage, binary activity outcome, control arm

A Practical Guide to Designing Phase II Trials in Oncology, First Edition.
Sarah R. Brown, Walter M. Gregory, Chris Twelves and Julia Brown.
© 2014 John Wiley & Sons, Ltd. Published 2014 by John Wiley & Sons, Ltd.

- Formal comparison with control

- Requires programming

Thall and Cheng outline a randomised controlled design to assess safety and activity as a bivariate variable, quantifying treatment effect as a corresponding two-dimensional parameter. The design considers the acceptable trade-off in toxicity for increases in activity, that is, the acceptable increase in toxicity for a specific increase in activity, and vice versa, and provides a formal comparison of the experimental treatment with control. It is necessary to specify the control activity and toxicity estimates and trade-offs that would be acceptable to warrant the experimental treatment worthy of further investigation; more than one trade-off can be specified. The association between toxicity and activity should also be specified in terms of an odds ratio (OR) between the probability of toxicity when, for example, response occurs, relative to no response, where an OR of 1 implies independence between toxicity and response. The design presented is a one-stage design and is extended to multiple stages in a subsequent paper (Thall and Cheng 2001). Programs are not detailed as being available; however, detail is given to allow implementation, and programs may be available by contacting the authors.

6.1.1.2   Time-to-event outcome measure

Thall and Cheng (1999)

- One-stage, time-to-event activity outcome, control arm

- Formal comparison with control

- Requires programming

- No early termination

Thall and Cheng outline a randomised controlled design to assess safety and activity as a bivariate variable, quantifying treatment effect as a corresponding two-dimensional parameter. The design considers the acceptable trade-off in toxicity for increases in activity, that is, the acceptable increase in toxicity for a specific increase in activity, and vice versa, and provides a formal comparison of the experimental treatment with control. It is necessary to specify the control activity and toxicity estimates and trade-offs that would be acceptable to warrant the experimental treatment worthy of further investigation; more than one trade-off can be specified. The association between toxicity and activity should also be specified. The main body of the paper outlines the design in the context of a binary outcome for activity; however, distribution theory for application with a time-to-event outcome is provided in the appendix to the paper. The design presented is a one-stage design and is extended to multiple stages in a subsequent paper (Thall and Cheng 2001). Programs are not detailed as being available; however, detail is given to allow implementation, and programs may be available by contacting the authors.

6.1.2   Two-stage designs

6.1.2.1   Binary outcome measure

Thall and Cheng (2001)

- Two-stage, binary activity outcome, control arm

- Formal comparison with control

- Requires programming

- Early termination for lack of activity or unacceptably high toxicity

Thall and Cheng extend the one-stage design outlined in Section 6.1.1 to the two-stage and multi-stage settings (Thall and Cheng 1999). The design considers the acceptable trade-offs in toxicity for increases in activity, that is, the acceptable increase in toxicity for a specific increase in activity, and vice versa, and provides a formal comparison of the experimental treatment with control. It is necessary to specify the control activity and toxicity estimates and trade-offs that would be acceptable to warrant the experimental treatment worthy of further investigation; more than one trade-off can be specified. The association between toxicity and activity should also be specified in terms of an OR between the probability of toxicity when, for example, response occurs, relative to no response, where an OR of 1 implies independence between toxicity and response. Sample size is either minimised under the null hypothesis of no treatment difference in activity and toxicity or the maximum sample size is minimised if the trial continues to a second stage. In the two-stage setting, termination at the end of stage 1 is permitted only for lack of activity or unacceptably high toxicity. The authors also discuss application to the single-arm phase II setting. No software is noted; however, detail is given to allow implementation.

Sun et al. (2009)

- Two-stage, binary activity outcome, control arm

- Formal comparison with control

- Software noted as being available from author

- Early termination for lack of activity or unacceptably high toxicity

Sun and colleagues propose a randomised two-stage design for activity as the primary outcome of a phase II trial, whereby a sufficiently high response rate *or* a sufficiently low early progressive disease rate should warrant further investigation of the treatment. This is assessed as a multinomial outcome. As such, the authors note that the design may be extended to studies monitoring safety and efficacy simultaneously. In this setting, the activity outcome may be considered as a binary outcome measure. Optimal and minimax designs are proposed following the methodology of Simon (1989). Differences in response and toxicity rates between control and experimental arms are compared, highlighting that the intention of the phase II trial is to screen for potential efficacy as opposed to identifying statistically significant differences. Decision rules are based on observing a sufficiently high response rate *or* a sufficiently low toxicity rate. An extension is also proposed to the multi-arm selection setting. Detail is given regarding how to implement the designs in practice, and software is noted as being available by contacting the first author to allow identification of designs. The design recommends a treatment for further investigation when the response rate is sufficiently high or the toxicity rate is sufficiently low. Early termination is permitted for lack of activity or unacceptably high toxicity only.

6.1.2.2   Time-to-event outcome measure

Thall and Cheng (2001)

- Two-stage, time-to-event activity outcome, control arm

- Formal comparison with control

- Requires programming

- Early termination for lack of activity or unacceptably high toxicity

Thall and Cheng extend the one-stage design outlined in Section 6.1.1 to the two-stage and multi-stage setting (Thall and Cheng 1999). The design considers the acceptable trade-offs in toxicity for increases in activity, that is, the acceptable increase in toxicity for a specific increase in activity, and vice versa, and provides a formal comparison of the experimental treatment with control. It is necessary to specify the control activity and toxicity estimates and trade-offs that would be acceptable to warrant the experimental treatment worthy of further investigation; more than one trade-off can be specified. The association between toxicity and activity should also be specified. The example provided by the authors outlines the design in the context of a binary outcome for activity; however, distribution theory provided for the one-stage design may be applied for application in the setting of a time-to-event outcome for activity (Thall and Cheng 1999). In the two-stage setting, termination at the end of stage 1 is permitted only for lack of activity or unacceptably high toxicity. The authors also discuss application to the single-arm phase II setting. No software is noted; however, detail is given to allow implementation.

6.1.3   Multi-stage designs

6.1.3.1   Binary outcome measure

Thall and Cheng (2001)

- Multi-stage, binary activity outcome, control arm

- Formal comparison with control

- Requires programming

- Early termination for lack of activity or unacceptable toxicity, or early termination for activity and acceptable toxicity

Thall and Cheng extend the one-stage design outlined in Section 6.1.1 to the two-stage and multi-stage setting (Thall and Cheng 1999). The design considers the acceptable trade-offs in toxicity for increases in activity, that is, the acceptable increase in toxicity for a specific increase in activity, and vice versa, and provides a formal comparison of the experimental treatment with control. It is necessary to specify the control activity and toxicity estimates and trade-offs that would be acceptable to warrant the experimental treatment worthy of further investigation; more than one trade-off can be specified. The association between toxicity and activity should also be specified in terms of an OR between the probability of toxicity when, for example, response occurs, relative to no response, where an OR of 1 implies independence between toxicity and response. In the multi-stage setting, termination at each interim assessment is permitted either for rejection of the alternative hypothesis (i.e. unacceptable toxicity or lack of activity) or for rejection of the null hypothesis (i.e. acceptable toxicity and activity). The authors also discuss application to the single-arm phase II setting. No software is noted; however, detail is given to allow implementation.

6.1.3.2   Time-to-event outcome measure

Thall and Cheng (2001)

- Multi-stage, time-to-event activity outcome, control arm

- Formal comparison with control

- Requires programming

- Early termination for lack of activity or unacceptably high toxicity or early termination for activity and acceptable toxicity

Thall and Cheng extend the one-stage design outlined in Section 6.1.1 to the two-stage and multi-stage setting (Thall and Cheng 1999). The design considers the acceptable trade-offs in toxicity for increases in activity, that is, the acceptable increase in toxicity for a specific increase in activity, and vice versa, and provides a formal comparison of the experimental treatment with control. It is necessary to specify the control activity and toxicity estimates and trade-offs that would be acceptable to warrant the experimental treatment worthy of further investigation; more than one trade-off can be specified. The association between toxicity and activity should also be specified. The example provided by the authors outlines the design in the context of a binary outcome for activity; however, distribution theory provided for the one-stage design may be applied for application in the setting of a time-to-event outcome for activity (Thall and Cheng 1999). In the multi-stage setting, termination at each interim assessment is permitted either for rejection of the alternative hypothesis (i.e. unacceptable toxicity or lack of activity) or for rejection of the null hypothesis (i.e. acceptable toxicity and activity). The authors also discuss application to the single-arm phase II setting. No software is noted; however, detail is given to allow implementation.

6.2   Not including a control arm

6.2.1   One-stage designs

6.2.1.1   Binary outcome measure

Conaway and Petroni (1995)

- One-stage, binary activity outcome, no control

- Programs noted as being available from authors

Conaway and Petroni propose a single-arm, bivariate outcome design for use when the sample size is limited to a small number of patients. The design considers both response and toxicity (both binary variables) and may be one-stage, two-stage or multi-stage. Estimation of the association between the activity and toxicity outcomes is required, for example, in the form of the correlation or an OR between the probability of toxicity when, for example, response occurs, relative to no response, where an OR of 1 implies independence between toxicity and response. The authors note that the design, with respect to power, is robust against misspecification of this association parameter. Sample sizes and cut-off points are calculated via iteration to satisfy the error criteria, and generally group sizes of fewer than 10 are not considered. Programs to enable implementation are noted as being available from the authors.

Conaway and Petroni (1996)

- One-stage, binary activity outcome, no control

- Requires programming

Conaway and Petroni propose a single-stage (and a two-stage) design for a single-arm trial in which both toxicity and activity (with reference to a response outcome) are incorporated. A trade-off between the two outcomes, that is, the acceptable increase in toxicity for a specific increase in activity, and vice versa, is incorporated based on the I-divergence test statistic. Four outcomes are assumed (active/not toxic; active/toxic; not active/toxic; not active/not toxic). The minimum response rate acceptable if there were no toxicities and the maximum toxicity rate acceptable if there was 100% response are required to be specified, as well as the OR for the dependence between the two outcomes, that is, the probability of toxicity when response occurs, relative to no response, where an OR of 1 implies independence between toxicity and response. To determine the total sample sizes and the cut-off boundaries iteration is required, where the cut-offs are based on the I-divergence test statistic. The authors recommend that, in practice, several values of the OR be investigated to assess the sensitivity of the design to misspecification in each setting. The authors note that the properties of the design are generally unaffected by misspecification. This design differs from their previous design (Conaway and Petroni 1995) which bases results on the overall activity and toxicity rates, as opposed to considering the four outcomes described above. Programs are not noted as being available from the authors; therefore, the design may need programming for implementation.

Jin (2007)

- One-stage, binary activity outcome, no control

- Requires programming

Jin considers a single-stage design incorporating both activity and toxicity as binary outcome measures, with extension to the two-stage setting. The design allows a trade-off between toxicity and activity by controlling the marginal type I errors for these two outcomes separately. Incorporating this additional control inevitably increases sample size. There are four potential outcomes: active/not toxic; active/toxic; not active/toxic; not active/not toxic which are summarised by means of specification of the overall response rate and overall toxicity rate, as well as the OR representing the association between the two, that is, the probability of toxicity when response occurs, relative to no response, where an OR of 1 implies independence between toxicity and response. The design is noted to be robust against misspecification of this OR. This design would need programming to enable implementation.

6.2.2   Two-stage designs

6.2.2.1   Binary outcome measure

Bryant and Day (1995)

- Two-stage, binary activity outcome, no control

- Standard software available

- Early termination for lack of activity or unacceptably high toxicity

Bryant and Day propose a two-stage, single-arm design that incorporates both toxicity and activity as binary outcome variables, in a design that reflects that of Simon's two-stage design for a single outcome (Simon 1989). Tables are presented for specific design scenarios, with further designs accessible via available software (Machin et al. 2008). Early termination is permitted for unacceptably low activity or unacceptably high toxicity only. The design assumes toxicity and activity are independent; this is arguably unlikely to be the case for most trials; however, the impact of incorrectly assuming independence was assessed and the design found to be reasonably insensitive to this. Additionally Tournoux et al. (2007) note that this design is more robust to misspecification of the relationship between toxicity and activity than that proposed by Conaway and Petroni (1995).

Conaway and Petroni (1995)

- Two-stage, binary activity outcome, no control

- Programs noted as being available from authors

- Early termination for lack of activity or unacceptably high toxicity

Conaway and Petroni propose a single-arm, bivariate outcome design for use when the sample size is limited to a small number of patients. The design considers both response and toxicity (both binary variables) and may be one-stage, two-stage or multi-stage. Estimation of the association between the activity and toxicity outcomes is required, for example, in the form of the correlation or an OR between the probability of toxicity when, for example, response occurs, relative to no response, where an OR of 1 implies independence between toxicity and response. The authors note that the design, with respect to power, is robust against misspecification of this association parameter. Sample sizes and cut-off points are calculated via iteration to satisfy the error criteria, and generally group sizes of fewer than 10 are not considered. Programs to enable implementation are noted as being available from the authors. In the two-stage design, the trial may terminate for lack of activity or unacceptable toxicity only, at the end of the first stage.

Conaway and Petroni (1996)

- Two-stage, binary activity outcome, no control

- Requires programming

- Early termination for lack of activity or unacceptably high toxicity

Conaway and Petroni propose a two-stage (and one-stage) design for a single-arm trial in which both toxicity and activity (with reference to a response outcome) are incorporated. A trade-off between the two outcomes, that is, the acceptable increase in toxicity for a specific increase in activity, and vice versa, is incorporated based on the I-divergence test statistic. Four outcomes are assumed (active/not toxic; active/toxic; not active/toxic; not active/not toxic). The minimum response rate acceptable if there were no toxicities and the maximum toxicity rate acceptable if there was 100% response are required to be specified, as well as the OR for the dependence between the two outcomes, that is, the probability of toxicity when response occurs, relative to no response, where an OR of 1 implies independence between toxicity and response. To determine the total sample sizes and the cut-off boundaries iteration is required, where the cut-offs are based on the I-divergence test statistic. The authors recommend that, in practice, several values of the OR be investigated to assess the sensitivity of the design to misspecification in each setting. The authors note that the properties of the design are generally unaffected by misspecification. This design differs from their previous design (Conaway and Petroni 1995) which bases results on the overall activity and toxicity rates, as opposed to considering the four outcomes described above. Programs are not noted as being available from the authors; therefore, the design may need programming for implementation.

Thall and Cheng (2001)

- Two-stage, binary activity outcome, no control
- Requires programming
- Early termination for lack of activity or unacceptably high toxicity

Thall and Cheng propose a two-stage design incorporating a control arm, which may be extended to the setting of a single-arm phase II trial incorporating both activity and toxicity. The design considers the acceptable trade-offs in toxicity for increases in activity, that is, the acceptable increase in toxicity for a specific increase in activity, and vice versa. It is necessary to specify the historical control activity and toxicity estimates and trade-offs that would be acceptable to warrant the experimental treatment worthy of further investigation. The association between toxicity and activity should also be specified. Termination at the end of the first stage is for lack of activity or unacceptable toxicity only. The procedure is generalised such that the hypothesis that the experimental treatment provides an improvement in activity and no increase in the toxicity rate may be considered; this differs form other designs that assume an improvement in both outcomes. No software is detailed; therefore, this design would need to be programmed to enable implementation.

Jin (2007)

- Two-stage, binary activity outcome, no control
- Requires programming
- Early termination for lack of activity or unacceptably high toxicity

Jin describes a one-stage design incorporating both activity and toxicity as binary outcome measures, with extension to the two-stage setting. The design allows a trade-off between toxicity and activity by controlling the marginal type I errors for these two outcomes separately. Incorporating this additional control inevitably increases sample size. There are four potential outcomes: active/not toxic; active/toxic; not active/toxic; not active/not toxic which are summarised by means of specification of the overall response rate and overall toxicity rate, as well as the OR representing the association between the two, that is, the probability of toxicity when response occurs, relative to no response, where an OR of 1 implies independence between toxicity and response. The design is noted to be robust against misspecification of this OR. This design would need programming to enable implementation. In the two-stage design, early termination is permitted for lack of activity or unacceptable toxicity.

Wu and Liu (2007)

- Two-stage, binary activity outcome, no control

- Sample size calculation as per other designs

- Early termination based on sample size re-estimation

Wu and Liu describe an adaptation to traditional designs incorporating both toxicity and activity as binary outcome measures (e.g. Conaway and Petroni 1995). The adaptation takes into account the possibility of misspecification of the OR for the probability of toxicity when response occurs, relative to no response. The overall sample size is calculated based on this OR, following the methods of previous designs such as Conaway and Petroni (1995), using an initial estimate of the OR. An interim assessment is performed after n_1 patients, chosen arbitrarily, at which point a sample size re-estimation is performed based on the observed OR for these patients. In this design, the purpose of the interim assessment is for sample size re-estimation only, and the design does not incorporate early termination for lack of activity or unacceptable toxicity at this stage. Type I and II errors are controlled and the trial may be terminated at the end of the first stage if the re-estimated sample size (n_{new}) is less than that of the initial stage (i.e. $n_{new} \leq n_1$). Programming requirements follow the methods used to determine initial sample size with calculation of the OR at the end of the first stage to re-estimate sample size.

6.2.2.2   Time-to-event outcome measure

Thall and Cheng (2001)

- Two-stage, time-to-event activity outcome, no control

- Requires programming

- Early termination for lack of activity or unacceptably high toxicity

Thall and Cheng propose a two-stage design incorporating a control arm, which may be extended to the setting of a single-arm phase II trial incorporating both activity and toxicity. The design considers the acceptable trade-offs in toxicity for increases in activity, that is, the acceptable increase in toxicity for a specific increase in activity, and vice versa. It is necessary to specify the historical control activity and toxicity estimates and trade-offs that would be acceptable to warrant the experimental treatment worthy of further investigation. The association between toxicity and activity should also be specified. The procedure is generalised such that the hypothesis that the experimental treatment provides an improvement in activity and no increase in the toxicity rate may be considered; this differs from other designs that assume an improvement in both outcomes. The example provided by the authors outlines the design in the context of a binary outcome for activity; however, distribution theory provided for the one-stage design may be applied for application in the setting of a time-to-event outcome for activity (Thall and Cheng 1999). No software is detailed;

therefore, this design would need to be programmed to enable implementation. In the two-stage design early termination at the end of stage 1 is permitted only for lack of activity or unacceptably high toxicity.

6.2.3   Multi-stage designs

6.2.3.1   Binary outcome measure

Conaway and Petroni (1995)

- Multi-stage, binary activity outcome, no control

- Programs noted as being available from authors

- Early termination for lack of activity or unacceptably high toxicity

Conaway and Petroni propose a single-arm, bivariate outcome design for use when the sample size is limited to a small number of patients. The design considers both response and toxicity (both binary variables) and may be one-stage, two-stage or multi-stage. Estimation of the association between the activity and toxicity outcomes is required, for example, in the form of the correlation or an OR between the probability of toxicity when, for example, response occurs, relative to no response, where an OR of 1 implies independence between toxicity and response. The authors note that the design, with respect to power, is robust against misspecification of this association parameter. Sample sizes and cut-off points are calculated via iteration to satisfy the error criteria, and generally group sizes of fewer than 10 are not considered. Programs to enable implementation are noted as being available from the authors. In the multi-stage design, the trial may terminate for lack of activity or unacceptable toxicity only, at the end of each stage.

Thall et al. (1996)

- Multi-stage, binary activity outcome, no control

- Programs noted as being available from author

- Early termination for lack of activity or unacceptably high toxicity

Thall and colleagues outline a Bayesian multi-stage (or continuous monitoring) design that considers both toxicity and activity in a single-arm trial, based on trade-offs in toxicity for increased activity. Patients are considered to have one of four possible outcomes (activity/no toxicity; activity/toxicity; no activity/no toxicity; no activity/toxicity). The posterior distribution for the experimental treatment is updated after every stage, and the trial may be terminated early for lack of activity or unacceptable toxicity. Stopping rules are presented graphically for the example presented within the paper. Simulation is used to determine the operating characteristics of the design, including the probability of early termination and the sample size distribution. Although the design requires group-sequential monitoring (or continuous monitoring), software is noted as being available upon request from the first author, which provides all the information to design and implement the trial.

Thall and Sung (1998)

- Multi-stage, binary activity outcome, no control
- Programs available on web
- Early termination for lack of activity or unacceptably high toxicity

Thall and Sung propose a Bayesian design that allows incorporation of multiple outcomes, specifically toxicity and activity, which is an extension of the design proposed by Thall et al. (1995). Extensions include the design of a phase II equivalence trial, whereby the phase II trial only requires to show that the experimental treatment is no worse than the historical control data and that there is at least some possibility of subsequently establishing confirmatory equivalence, or superiority, in a phase III trial. Outcomes are categorised into k levels (e.g. toxicity, response; toxicity, no response; no toxicity, response; no toxicity, no response). Dirichlet prior information for each of the k levels is used to design the trial, and software is available at http://bio statistics.mdanderson.org/SoftwareDownload/SingleSoftware.aspx?Software_Id=3 (last accessed June 2013).

Thall and Cheng (2001)

- Multi-stage, binary activity outcome, no control
- Requires programming
- Early termination for lack of activity or unacceptably high toxicity or early termination for activity and acceptable toxicity

Thall and Cheng propose a multi-stage design incorporating a control arm, which may be extended to the setting of a single-arm phase II trial incorporating both activity and toxicity. The design considers the acceptable trade-offs in toxicity for increases in activity, that is, the acceptable increase in toxicity for a specific increase in activity, and vice versa. It is necessary to specify the historical control activity and toxicity estimates and trade-offs that would be acceptable to warrant the experimental treatment worthy of further investigation. The association between toxicity and activity should also be specified. In the multi-stage setting, termination at each interim assessment is permitted either for rejection of the alternative hypothesis (i.e. unacceptable toxicity or lack of activity) or for rejection of the null hypothesis (i.e. acceptable toxicity and activity). The procedure is generalised such that the hypothesis that the experimental treatment provides an improvement in activity and no increase in the toxicity rate may be considered; this differs from other designs that assume an improvement in both outcomes. No software is detailed; therefore, this design would need to be programmed to enable implementation.

Thall et al. (2003)

- Multi-stage, binary activity outcome, no control

- Programs noted as being available from authors

- Early termination for lack of activity or unacceptably high toxicity

Thall and colleagues propose a hierarchical Bayesian design to investigate multiple disease sub-types in a single-arm trial (described in Chapter 7), for which detail is given to extend this to incorporate both toxicity and activity outcome measures. The design incorporates the probabilities of four possible outcomes: activity/no toxicity; activity/toxicity; no activity/no toxicity; no activity/toxicity. Differing treatment effects may be targeted within differing disease sub-types. Data observed in each subgroup of patients are used to provide information across all subgroups, thus 'sharing' data to update the posterior distributions across multiple disease sub-types. The trial may be terminated early for lack of activity or unacceptable toxicity. Simulation is required to update the posterior distribution after every group of patients; therefore, the design is computationally intensive. Programs are noted as being available upon request from the authors to allow simulation, and programs for computing stopping boundaries are provided in the appendix to the manuscript.

6.2.3.2   Time-to-event outcome measure

Thall and Cheng (2001)

- Multi-stage, time-to-event activity outcome, no control

- Requires programming

- Early termination for lack of activity or unacceptably high toxicity or early termination for activity and acceptable toxicity

Thall and Cheng propose a multi-stage design incorporating a control arm, which may be extended to the setting of a single-arm phase II trial incorporating both activity and toxicity. The design considers the acceptable trade-offs in toxicity for increases in activity, that is, the acceptable increase in toxicity for a specific increase in activity, and vice versa. It is necessary to specify the historical control activity and toxicity estimates and trade-offs that would be acceptable to warrant the experimental treatment worthy of further investigation. The association between toxicity and activity should also be specified. The procedure is generalised such that the hypothesis that the experimental treatment provides an improvement in activity and no increase in the toxicity rate may be considered; this differs from other designs that assume an improvement in both outcomes. The example provided by the authors outlines the design in the context of a binary outcome for activity; however, distribution theory provided for the one-stage design may be applied for application in the setting of a time-to-event outcome for activity (Thall and Cheng 1999). No software is detailed; therefore, this design would need to be programmed to enable implementation. In the multi-stage setting, termination at each interim assessment is permitted either for rejection of the alternative hypothesis (i.e. unacceptable toxicity or lack of activity) or for rejection of the null hypothesis (i.e. acceptable toxicity and activity).

6.2.4   Continuous monitoring designs

6.2.4.1   Binary outcome measure

Thall et al. (1996)

- Continuous monitoring, binary activity outcome, no control
- Programs noted as being available from author
- Early termination for lack of activity or unacceptably high toxicity

Thall and colleagues outline a Bayesian continuous monitoring (or multi-stage) design that considers both toxicity and activity in a single-arm trial, based on trade-offs in toxicity for increased activity. Patients are considered to have one of four possible outcomes (activity/no toxicity; activity/toxicity; no activity/no toxicity; no activity/toxicity). The posterior distribution for the experimental treatment is updated continuously after every stage, and the trial may be terminated early for lack of activity or unacceptable toxicity. Stopping rules are presented graphically for the example presented within the paper. Simulation is used to determine the operating characteristics of the design, including the probability of early termination and the sample size distribution. Although the design requires continuous monitoring (or group-sequential monitoring), software is noted as being available upon request from the first author, which provides all the information to design and implement the trial.

Thall and Sung (1998)

- Continuous monitoring, binary activity outcome, no control
- Programs available on web
- Early termination for lack of activity or unacceptably high toxicity

Thall and Sung propose a Bayesian design that allows incorporation of multiple outcomes, specifically toxicity and activity, which is an extension of the design proposed by Thall et al. (1995). Extensions include the design of a phase II equivalence trial, whereby the phase II trial only requires to show that the experimental treatment is no worse than the historical control data and that there is at least some possibility of subsequently establishing confirmatory equivalence, or superiority, in a phase III trial. Outcomes are categorised into k levels (e.g. toxicity, response; toxicity, no response; no toxicity, response; no toxicity, no response). Dirichlet prior information for each of the k levels is used to design the trial, and software is available at http://bio statistics.mdanderson.org/SoftwareDownload/SingleSoftware.aspx?Software_Id=3 (last accessed June 2013).

Thall et al. (2003)

- Continuous monitoring, binary activity outcome, no control
- Programs noted as being available from authors
- Early termination for lack of activity or unacceptably high toxicity

Thall and colleagues propose a hierarchical Bayesian design to investigate multiple disease sub-types in a single-arm trial (described in Chapter 7), for which detail is given to extend this to incorporate both toxicity and activity outcome measures. The design incorporates the probabilities of four possible outcomes: activity/ no toxicity; activity/toxicity; no activity/no toxicity; no activity/toxicity. Differing treatment effects may be targeted within differing disease sub-types. Data observed in each subgroup of patients are used to provide information across all subgroups, thus 'sharing' data to update the posterior distributions across multiple disease sub-types. The trial may be terminated early for lack of activity or unacceptable toxicity. Simulation is required to update the posterior distribution after every group of patients; therefore, the design is computationally intensive. Programs are noted as being available upon request from the authors to allow simulation, and programs for computing stopping boundaries are provided in the appendix to the manuscript.

6.3   Toxicity alone

6.3.1   One stage

de Boo and Zielhuis (2004)

- One-stage, binary toxicity outcome, control arm
- Formal comparison with control
- Programs noted as being available from authors
- No early termination

de Boo and Zielhuis propose sample size calculations for single-stage, non-inferiority trials of safety where toxicity probabilities are small. This design considers toxicity alone and may be incorporated as an add-on to a trial designed to assess activity, with toxicity assessed at the end of the trial. Details of computation are given in the appendix of the manuscript, and a SAS program is noted as being available upon request from the authors. Formal comparison between the experimental and control arms is incorporated. Due to small toxicity probabilities and formal comparison, the design can require large numbers of patients. Operating characteristics may be investigated to assess design performance when incorporated as an add-on to an activity trial (i.e. where sample size is determined according to the design of the activity trial).

6.3.2 Continuous monitoring

Goldman (1987)

- Continuous monitoring, binary toxicity outcome, no control

- Requires programming

- Early termination for unacceptably high toxicity

Goldman proposes stopping rules when monitoring toxicities (as a binary outcome) in a single-arm, small study. The sequential probability ratio test (SPRT) is used to calculate stopping rules as a function of the number of patients and events (toxicities), to give a design of the form $(-,a,b,c,\ldots h)$ which is interpreted as follows: the trial should not stop after just one toxicity, but would stop if two toxicities were observed in a patients, three in b patients, ... up to nine toxicities in h number of patients. The design considers stopping boundaries of toxicity only and should be adapted to ensure that the operating characteristics of the design are as close to the required values as possible. Programming is therefore required to implement this; however, it is noted that a program has been written, therefore this may be available upon request. The author notes that this design is only relevant for small, single-sample studies when early termination is for an excess of toxicities only. For studies with large fixed sample sizes, or multiple outcome testing, probabilities of early termination may be better calculated using Monte Carlo simulation.

Goldman and Hannan (2001)

- Continuous monitoring, binary toxicity outcome, no control

- Programs noted as being available from authors and on web

- Early termination for unacceptably high toxicity

Goldman and Hannan propose a continuous monitoring design that considers the toxicity of a treatment and runs alongside a single-arm design for activity (i.e. this is an add-on), as an adaptation to the earlier design of Goldman, described above (Goldman 1987). It assumes activity is *not* continuously monitored. Sample size is determined as per the primary activity design, and stopping rules for toxicity are generated based on sample size, null and alternative toxicity rates and type I error. A FORTRAN program is noted as being available from the authors to identify the design. The design is of the form $(-,a,b,c,\ldots,h)$ which is interpreted as follows: the trial should not stop after just one toxicity, but would stop if two toxicities were observed in a patients, three in b patients, ... up to nine toxicities in h number of patients (as in the design described above). This design uses the original 1987 paper and incorporates the algorithm into a larger FORTRAN program which also outputs the average sample number (accounting for the possibility of early termination). This is available at http://www.biostat.umn.edu/Projects/bounds/ (last accessed July 2013). Evaluation takes place whenever toxicity occurs, and the authors note that the design performs well in up to 20–30 patients. This approach does not consider the effect on the activity assumptions due to the additional toxicity monitoring, unlike the design proposed by Ivanova et al. (2005; described below).

Ivanova et al. (2005)

- Continuous monitoring, binary toxicity outcome, no control

- Programs available on web

- Early termination for unacceptably high toxicity

Ivanova and colleagues propose a continuous monitoring design for toxicity that can be added on to a single-stage design for activity. Stopping boundaries are created to assess toxicity after every patient and stop the trial early in the case of extreme toxicity. Although the toxicity outcome does not need to be observed before the next patient can be recruited, it does need to be monitored in real time as analysis is performed after every patient. A fixed sample size calculated as per the primary activity design is required to calculate the stopping boundaries for toxicity. If the trial does not stop early for toxicity then the decision criteria for phase III are based on the activity outcome at the end of the trial. Outcomes of toxicity and response are binary, and details of estimation of toxicity and response rates are given, for which the correlation between the two outcome measures is required. These need to be considered at the design stage as the evaluation of toxicity may result in bias of the estimate of response. It is noted that unless toxicity and activity are highly correlated, there is little effect on the estimate of response obtained by incorporating an additional toxicity assessment. This design differs from that described by Goldman (1987) in that it uses O'Brien and Fleming or Pocock stopping boundaries (O'Brien and Fleming 1979; Pocock 1977) instead of the SPRT (which assumes open-ended samples) and considers calculation of unbiased estimates of toxicity and response. Software to identify the design is available from http://www.bios.unc.edu/distrib/gee/crossing/cp3/ (last accessed July 2013).

6.4   Treatment selection based on activity and toxicity

6.4.1   Two-stage designs

Sun et al. (2009)

- Two-stage, activity and toxicity, control arm

- Formally powered statistical comparison between arms

- Software noted as being available from author

- Early termination for lack of activity or unacceptably high toxicity

Sun and colleagues propose a randomised two-stage design based on Zee's single-arm multi-stage design with multinomial outcome measure (Zee et al. 1999). It is noted that the design may be extended to studies monitoring safety and efficacy simultaneously. Decision rules are based on observing a sufficiently high response rate *or* a sufficiently low toxicity rate. Optimal and minimax designs are proposed following the methodology of Simon (1989). Differences in response and toxicity between control and experimental arms are compared, with the intention of screening for potential efficacy as opposed to identifying statistically significant differences. Patients are randomised between multiple experimental treatments and a control arm. At the end of the first stage only those treatments that pass the stopping boundaries for both response and toxicity are continued to the second stage. If there is clear evidence that one treatment is better than the other, selection may take place at the end of the first stage. If, at the end of the second stage, there is no clear evidence that one experimental treatment is better than the other, both arms may be considered for further evaluation. Detail is given regarding how to implement the designs in practice, and software is noted as being available by contacting the first author to allow identification of designs.

6.4.2   Multi-stage designs

Thall and Sung (1998)

- Multi-stage, activity and toxicity, no control arm

- No formal comparison between arms

- Programs available on web

- Early termination for lack of activity or unacceptably high toxicity

Thall and Sung propose a Bayesian design that allows incorporation of multiple outcomes, specifically toxicity and activity, which is noted to be an extension of Thall et al. (1995). Designs can be single arm or multi-arm for treatment selection. The outcomes are categorised into k levels (e.g. toxicity, response; toxicity, no response; no toxicity, response; no toxicity, no response). Dirichlet prior information for each of the k levels is used to design the trial, and software is available at http://bio statistics.mdanderson.org/SoftwareDownload/SingleSoftware.aspx?Software_Id=3 (last accessed June 2013). Treatment selection is based on the approaches of Simon et al. (1985) and Thall and Estey (1993), such that the treatment with, for example, the highest response rate is correctly selected with a pre-specified minimum probability. It is noted that it does take considerably more time to elicit the required information for this design from clinicians than more standard designs; however, once this has been established, the design reflects a realistic representation of scientific and clinical requirements.

6.4.3   Continuous monitoring designs

Thall and Sung (1998)

- Continuous monitoring, activity and toxicity, no control arm

- No formal comparison between arms

- Programs available on web

- Early termination for lack of activity or unacceptably high toxicity

Thall and Sung propose a Bayesian design that allows incorporation of multiple outcomes, specifically toxicity and activity, which is noted to be an extension of Thall et al. (1995). Designs can be single arm or multi-arm for treatment selection. An adaptation to the multi-stage design can be made to allow continuous monitoring. The outcomes are categorised into k levels (e.g. toxicity, response; toxicity, no response; no toxicity, response; no toxicity, no response). Dirichlet prior information for each of the k levels is used to design the trial, and software is available at http://bio statistics.mdanderson.org/SoftwareDownload/SingleSoftware.aspx?Software_Id=3 (last accessed June 2013). Treatment selection is based on the approaches of Simon et al. (1985) and Thall and Estey (1993), such that the treatment with, for example, the highest response rate is correctly selected with a pre-specified minimum probability. It is noted that it does take considerably more time to elicit the required information for this design from clinicians than more standard designs; however, once this has been established, the design reflects a realistic representation of scientific and clinical requirements.

7

Designs evaluating targeted subgroups

Sarah Brown

This chapter summarises those designs identified via the literature review that may be used for the purpose of evaluating targeted subgroups of patients. As discussed previously, there have been a number of recently published articles in this area that have not been evaluated for inclusion here since they post-date the updated systematic review on which the library is based. Where the incorporation of biomarkers are of particular relevance to a trial design, the designs described within this chapter should be considered; however, we encourage further review of more recent designs specifically intended for trials incorporating biomarkers.

7.1 One-stage designs

7.1.1 Binary outcome measure

A'Hern (2004)

- One-stage, binary outcome

- No control arm incorporated

- Programs noted as being available from author

A'Hern outlines a single-arm, one-stage (and two-stage) design that takes into account differing response likelihoods for different subgroups of patients, based on

A Practical Guide to Designing Phase II Trials in Oncology, First Edition.
Sarah R. Brown, Walter M. Gregory, Chris Twelves and Julia Brown.
© 2014 John Wiley & Sons, Ltd. Published 2014 by John Wiley & Sons, Ltd.

the constant arcsine difference (CAD) between upper and lower response limits, which has a constant variance. Null and alternative outcomes are specified for each group and the CAD calculated and assumed constant across each group. In practice, one specifies the null and alternative hypothesis values for a known prognostic group, calculates the corresponding CAD and then calculates equivalent differences for other prognostic groups, considering whether or not these differences would be clinically realistic in other groups. Cut-off values for the distribution of CAD are calculated during the trial, requiring an algorithm to be updated after each patient (towards the end of recruitment), and therefore continuous monitoring is required. Programs are noted as being available from the author to run this in excel.

London and Chang (2005)

- One-stage, binary outcome

- No control arm incorporated

- Requires programming

London and Chang incorporate assessment of response rate within strata in their proposed design. Two approaches are proposed: one for which the true proportion of patients in each strata is assumed known (the unconditional approach) and one for which this is assumed unknown (the conditional approach). A simulation algorithm is provided to identify sample size and stopping rules for the unconditional approach, and exact computation is used for the conditional approach. Details are provided in the manuscript; however, both of the approaches will require programming. An estimate of the accrual rate to each stratum is required initially to determine sample size. If, during the course of the trial, the actual stratum proportions are very different to the estimates used, a sample size adjustment may be required during the trial. In general, the conditional approach is recommended, as an accurate estimate of the proportion of patients in each stratum is not required and it is noted to be robust to changes in the proportion of patients within each stratum if the observed proportions are not too far away from the expected proportions. If researchers are very unsure of the likely proportions, a number of differing proportions should be considered and the most conservative sample size taken.

7.2   Two-stage designs

7.2.1   Binary outcome measure

A'Hern (2004)

- Two-stage, binary outcome

- No control arm incorporated

- Programs noted as being available from author

- Early termination for lack of activity

A'Hern outlines a single-arm, two-stage (and one-stage) design that takes into account differing response likelihoods for different subgroups of patients, based on the CAD between upper and lower response limits, which has a constant variance. At the end of the first stage the trial may terminate early for lack of activity. Null and alternative outcomes are specified for each group and the CAD calculated and assumed constant across each group. In practice, one specifies the null and alternative hypothesis values for a known prognostic group, calculates the corresponding CAD and then calculates equivalent differences for other prognostic groups, considering whether or not these differences would be clinically realistic in other groups. Cut-off values for the distribution of CAD are calculated during the trial, requiring an algorithm to be updated after each patient (towards the end of recruitment), and therefore continuous monitoring is required. Programs are noted as being available from the author to run this in excel.

London and Chang (2005)

- Two-stage, binary outcome

- No control arm incorporated

- Requires programming

- Early termination for lack of activity

London and Chang incorporate assessment of response rate within strata in their proposed design. Two approaches are proposed: one for which the true proportion of patients in each strata is assumed known (the unconditional approach) and one for which this is assumed unknown (the conditional approach). A simulation algorithm is provided to identify sample size and stopping rules for the unconditional approach, and exact computation is used for the conditional approach. Details are provided in the manuscript; however, both of the approaches will require programming. An estimate of the accrual rate to each stratum is required initially to determine sample size. If, during the course of the trial, the actual stratum proportions are very different to the estimates used, a sample size adjustment may be required during the trial. In general, the conditional approach is recommended, as an accurate estimate of the proportion of patients in each stratum is not required and it is noted to be robust to changes in the proportion of patients within each stratum if the observed proportions are not too far away from the expected proportions. If researchers are very unsure of the likely proportions, a number of differing proportions should be considered and the most conservative sample size taken. For the two-stage unconditional approach the researcher is required to specify the proportion of the overall type I and type II error rates to be spent in the first stage. Additionally, early termination for lack of activity is permitted.

Pusztai et al. (2007)

- Two-stage, binary outcome

- No control arm incorporated

- Standard software available as per other designs
- Early termination for lack of activity

Pustzai and colleagues detail a single-arm two-stage design that considers the response to a single experimental treatment according to biomarker positivity. The goal is to determine whether the drug is likely to have a certain level of activity in unselected patients, and if it is below the level of interest at the end of the first stage, whether a particular patient selection method can enrich the responding population to meet the targeted level of activity in a molecularly selected group. The marker of interest needs to be specified before the trial begins, and more than one marker may be considered (and analyses conducted separately). Sample size and stopping boundaries are calculated as per other two-stage designs (e.g. Simon 1989). The trial is implemented as follows:

1. Recruit as normal to a traditional two-stage design, regardless of marker evaluation.

2. If at the end of stage 1 there are sufficient number of responses to continue to the next stage, continue as per traditional two-stage design, regardless of marker evaluation.

3. If at the end of stage 1 there are too few responses, continue the study in marker-positive patients only (there may be more than one marker under investigation), with an additional intermediate stage.

4. Assuming (3), if at the end of the next stage there are still too few responses, reject the drug for lack of activity, the marker has failed.

5. Assuming (3), if at the end of the next stage there are sufficient responses to justify continuation, continue to next stage in this group of patients.

6. Assuming (5), complete final stage of study to determine the activity of the drug in this subset of patients.

Jones and Holmgren (2007)

- Two-stage, binary outcome
- No control arm incorporated
- Standard software available
- Early termination for lack of activity

Jones and Holmgren outline a two-stage design, assuming a biomarker of interest is available at the start of the study and its prevalence is well established. It incorporates marker positivity/negativity in an adaptive Simon's two-stage design (Simon 1989). The authors initially describe a basic approach to assessing treatment activity in specific subgroups via two parallel two-stage designs. The adaptive parallel two-stage design proceeds as follows:

1. Begin with two parallel two-stage designs.

2. If, at the end of stage 1, the experimental treatment is deemed sufficiently active in both marker-positive and marker-negative subgroups, the trial continues on to the second stage in an unselected population.

3. If, at the end of stage 1, activity of the experimental treatment is restricted to only the marker-positive subgroup, the trial continues on to the second stage in marker-positive patients only.

As this design is an adapted Simon's two-stage design, software is available to calculate sample size and stopping boundaries, and early termination is permitted for lack of activity only. The design differs from that proposed by Pusztai et al. (2007) in that the biomarker and its prevalence are well established at the start of the trial, and the investigation is of one biomarker only, not many. Additionally the design considers marker-positive and marker-negative patients separately to begin with, whereas the design proposed by Pustzai et al. considers all patients initially, with grouping by marker positivity only if required.

7.3   Multi-stage designs

7.3.1   Binary outcome measure

Thall et al. (2003)

- Multi-stage, binary outcome

- No control arm incorporated

- Programs provided in appendix to manuscript, and further simulation programs noted as being available from authors

- Early termination for lack of activity

Thall and colleagues propose a hierarchical Bayesian design to investigate multiple disease sub-types in a single-arm trial. The design incorporates either a binary response outcome or a time-to-event outcome and may be conducted as either a multi-stage or continuous monitoring design, whereby stopping rules are applied at each assessment. Differing treatment effects may be targeted within differing disease sub-types. Data observed in each subgroup of patients are used to provide information across all subgroups, thus 'sharing' data to update the posterior distributions across multiple disease sub-types. The trial may be terminated early for lack of activity, and toxicity outcome measures may also be incorporated. Simulation is required to update the posterior distribution after every group of patients; therefore, the design is computationally intensive. Programs are noted as being available upon request from the authors to allow simulation, and programs for computing stopping boundaries are provided in the appendix to the manuscript.

Wathen et al. (2008)

- Multi-stage, binary outcome
- No control arm incorporated
- Programs may be available from authors
- Early termination for lack of activity

Wathen et al. outline a Bayesian design for single-arm multi-stage or continuous monitoring trials incorporating either a binary or time-to-event outcome and accounting for patient heterogeneity. The proposed design generalises the approaches of Thall et al. (2005) and Thall and Simon (1994b) using linear regression to incorporate a treatment–subgroup interaction. Treatment effects to be detected may differ between subgroups. Early termination for lack of activity is incorporated. The authors note that in the case where a treatment–subgroup interaction is unlikely to occur, simpler models may be sufficient and avoid the complexity of the proposed methodology. Simulations are required to validate the design with regard to the false-negative error rates and false-positive rates. The authors aim to provide free software for implementing the proposed method, which is assumed to be available from the authors.

Le Blanc et al. (2009)

- Multi-stage, binary outcome
- No control arm incorporated
- Standard software available
- Early termination for lack of activity

Le Blanc et al. outline a group-sequential design that allows incorporation of a wide population of patients when the specific target of a new drug is uncertain, such that hypothesis testing and analyses consider multiple subgroups of patients. Outcomes may be binary or the methodology adapted to time-to-event outcomes. Testing for lack of activity occurs within each stratum, or across all strata, when a pre-specified minimum number of patients have been accrued. Accrual may be terminated for lack of activity within a stratum or the whole trial may be terminated if the overall test for lack of activity is significant. This may also be adapted in the case where a specific subgroup is targeted as likely being the most active group, such that demonstrating lack of activity in this subgroup indicates terminating the study overall. Sample size calculations follow the two-stage design methodologies of Simon (1989), Korn et al. (2008) (to incorporate weighting) or Thall et al. (2003), to determine sample sizes within each stratum (total number of patients and minimum number of patients before testing for lack of activity should begin) and overall. Additionally, for time-to-event outcomes, large sample trials may follow the methodology of Lin et al. (1996) or evaluate small sample sizes via simulation.

7.3.2   Time-to-event outcome measure

Thall et al. (2003)

- Multi-stage, time-to-event outcome

- No control arm incorporated

- Programs provided in appendix to manuscript, and further simulation programs noted as being available from authors

- Early termination for lack of activity

Thall and colleagues propose a hierarchical Bayesian design to investigate multiple disease sub-types in a single-arm trial. The design incorporates either a binary response outcome or time-to-event outcome and may be conducted as either a multi-stage or continuous monitoring design, whereby stopping rules are applied at each assessment. Differing treatment effects may be targeted within differing disease sub-types. Data observed in each subgroup of patients are used to provide information across all subgroups, thus 'sharing' data to update the posterior distributions across multiple disease sub-types. The trial may be terminated early for lack of activity, and toxicity outcome measures may also be incorporated. Simulation is required to update the posterior distribution after every group of patients; therefore, the design is computationally intensive. Programs are noted as being available upon request from the authors to allow simulation, and programs for computing stopping boundaries are provided in the appendix to the manuscript.

Wathen et al. (2008)

- Multi-stage, time-to-event outcome

- No control arm incorporated

- Programs may be available from authors

- Early termination for lack of activity

Wathen et al. outline a Bayesian design for single-arm multi-stage or continuous monitoring trials incorporating either a binary or time-to-event outcome and accounting for patient heterogeneity. The proposed design generalises the approaches of Thall and Simon (1994b) and Thall et al. (2005), using linear regression to incorporate a treatment–subgroup interaction. Treatment effects to be detected may differ between subgroups. Early termination for lack of activity is incorporated. The authors note that in the case where a treatment–subgroup interaction is unlikely to occur, simpler models may be sufficient and avoid the complexity of the proposed methodology. Simulations are required to validate the design with regard to the false-negative error rates and false-positive rates. The authors aim to provide free software for implementing the proposed method, which is assumed to be available from the authors.

Le Blanc et al. (2009)

- Multi-stage, time-to-event outcome

- No control arm incorporated

- Standard software available

- Early termination for lack of activity

Le Blanc et al. outline a group-sequential design that allows incorporation of a wide population of patients when the specific target of a new drug is uncertain, such that hypothesis testing and analyses consider multiple subgroups of patients. Outcomes may be binary or the methodology adapted to time-to-event outcomes. Testing for lack of activity occurs within each stratum, or across all strata, when a pre-specified minimum number of patients have been accrued. Accrual may be terminated for lack of activity within a stratum or the whole trial may be terminated if the overall test for lack of activity is significant. This may also be adapted in the case where a specific subgroup is targeted as likely being the most active group, such that demonstrating lack of activity in this subgroup indicates terminating the study overall. Sample size calculations follow the two-stage design methodologies of Simon (1989), Korn et al. (2008) (to incorporate weighting) or Thall et al. (2003), to determine sample sizes within each stratum (total number of patients and minimum number of patients before testing for lack of activity should begin) and overall. Additionally, for time-to-event outcomes, large sample trials may follow the methodology of Lin et al. (1996) or evaluate small sample sizes via simulation.

7.4   Continuous monitoring designs

7.4.1   Binary outcome measure

Thall et al. (2003)

- Continuous monitoring, binary outcome

- No control arm incorporated

- Programs provided in appendix to manuscript, and further simulation programs noted as being available from authors

- Early termination for lack of activity

Thall and colleagues propose a hierarchical Bayesian design to investigate multiple disease sub-types in a single-arm trial. The design incorporates either a binary response outcome or time-to-event outcome and may be conducted as either a multi-stage or continuous monitoring design, whereby stopping rules are applied at each assessment. Differing treatment effects may be targeted within differing disease sub-types. Data observed in each subgroup of patients are used to provide information across all subgroups, thus 'sharing' data to update the posterior distributions across multiple disease sub-types. The trial may be terminated early for lack of activity and toxicity outcome measures may also be incorporated. Simulation is required to update the posterior distribution after every patient; therefore, the design is computationally intensive. Programs are noted as being available upon request from the authors to allow simulation, and programs for computing stopping boundaries are provided in the appendix to the manuscript.

Wathen et al. (2008)

- Continuous monitoring, binary outcome

- No control arm incorporated

- Programs may be available from authors

- Early termination for lack of activity

Wathen et al. outline a Bayesian design for single-arm multi-stage or continuous monitoring trials incorporating either a binary or time-to-event outcome and accounting for patient heterogeneity. The proposed design generalises the approaches of Thall and Simon (1994b) and Thall et al. (2005), using linear regression to incorporate a treatment–subgroup interaction. Treatment effects to be detected may differ between subgroups. Early termination for lack of activity is incorporated. The authors note that in the case where a treatment–subgroup interaction is unlikely to occur, simpler models may be sufficient and avoid the complexity of the proposed methodology. Simulations are required to validate the design with regard to the false-negative error rates and false-positive rates. The authors aim to provide free software for implementing the proposed method, which is assumed to be available from the authors.

7.4.2   Time-to-event outcome measure

Thall et al. (2003)

- Continuous monitoring, time-to-event outcome

- No control arm incorporated

- Programs provided in appendix to manuscript, and further simulation programs noted as being available from authors

- Early termination for lack of activity

Thall and colleagues propose a hierarchical Bayesian design to investigate multiple disease sub-types in a single-arm trial. The design incorporates either a binary response outcome or time-to-event outcome and may be conducted as either a multistage or continuous monitoring design, whereby stopping rules are applied at each assessment. Differing treatment effects may be targeted within differing disease sub-types. Data observed in each subgroup of patients are used to provide information across all subgroups, thus 'sharing' data to update the posterior distributions across multiple disease sub-types. The trial may be terminated early for lack of activity and toxicity outcome measures may also be incorporated. Simulation is required to update the posterior distribution after every patient; therefore, the design is computationally intensive. Programs are noted as being available upon request from the authors to allow simulation, and programs for computing stopping boundaries are provided in the appendix to the manuscript.

Wathen et al. (2008)

- Continuous monitoring, time-to-event outcome

- No control arm incorporated

- Programs may be available from authors

- Early termination for lack of activity

Wathen et al. outline a Bayesian design for single-arm multi-stage or continuous monitoring trials incorporating either a binary or time-to-event outcome and account-ing for patient heterogeneity. The proposed design generalises the approaches of Thall and Simon (1994b) and Thall et al. (2005), using linear regression to incorporate a treatment–subgroup interaction. Treatment effects to be detected may differ between subgroups. Early termination for lack of activity is incorporated. The authors note that in the case where a treatment–subgroup interaction is unlikely to occur, simpler models may be sufficient and avoid the complexity of the proposed methodology. Simulations are required to validate the design with regard to the false-negative error rates and false-positive rates. The authors aim to provide free software for imple-menting the proposed method, which is assumed to be available from the authors.

8

'Chemo-radio-sensitisation' in head and neck cancer

John Chester and Sarah Brown

Drug A is a molecularly-targeted cytostatic agent directed against Epidermal Growth Factor Receptor (EGFR), that was well tolerated as a single agent in phase I trials. It is hypothesised to enhance the efficacy of radiotherapy for patients presenting with locally-advanced head and neck squamous cell carcinoma (HNSCC), for whom current standard treatment is radiotherapy alone. The patient population size is relatively modest, but there are some historical data for treatment with radiotherapy alone, in this population. Data are also available from a patient population with more advanced disease in whom a previous phase III study with a similar molecularly-targeted agent demonstrated efficacy and an acceptable toxicity profile, when used in combination with radiotherapy. A phase II trial of drug A, in combination with radiotherapy as primary treatment, is proposed to be run as an academic study within a large collaborative group.

Stage 1 – Trial questions

Therapeutic considerations

Mechanism of action: Drug A is a molecularly-targeted cytostatic agent directed against EGFR. It is believed to be primarily cytostatic as a single agent, but to act synergistically with radiotherapy. It may therefore have both local radio-sensitising and systemic anti-tumour effects.

A Practical Guide to Designing Phase II Trials in Oncology, First Edition.
Sarah R. Brown, Walter M. Gregory, Chris Twelves and Julia Brown.

Aim of treatment: The ultimate aim of primary treatment for patients with locally-advanced disease is cure. Since the combination of drug A with radiotherapy may have both local and systemic anti-tumour effects, achieving radiological complete remission and remaining both locally and systemically disease-free are appropriate indicators of treatment activity.

Single or combination therapy: Drug A is given in combination with radiotherapy; therefore, any activity of the combination therapy would need to be greater than that of radiotherapy alone, the current standard treatment.

Biomarkers: There are no validated biomarkers associated with drug A or with HNSCC, to allow patient enrichment or surrogate assessment of therapeutic activity.

Primary intention of trial

Proof of concept data are available from an earlier phase III study of a similar agent in combination with radiotherapy, in the same tumour type, but in more advanced disease. Combination therapy was shown to be tolerable and achieved improved overall survival (OS) compared to radiotherapy alone in that setting. A proof of concept study for drug A in combination with radiotherapy is therefore not deemed necessary. Rather, the aim of the current trial is to make a go/no-go decision as to whether or not to proceed to a phase III trial of the combination in patients with locally-advanced HNSCC.

Number of experimental treatment arms

There is only one experimental treatment under investigation, so a treatment selection trial is not required.

Primary outcome of interest

Drug A has an acceptable toxicity profile in single-agent studies. Similar agents have been combined safely with radiotherapy in patients with more advanced disease, and therefore the current combination is expected to have only minimal additional toxicity or functional deficit. While toxicity will form a secondary endpoint of the phase II trial, the primary outcome of interest is activity.

Stage 2 – Design components

Outcome measure and distribution

Since drug A is a putative radio-sensitiser, the primary aim of combination with radiotherapy is to eliminate local disease and minimise disease recurrence. Event-free survival (EFS) is defined as the time from trial registration to first event (i.e. local or distant recurrence or death from any cause) and has been shown to be strongly correlated with OS in patients with locally-advanced HNSCC (Michiels et al. 2009). Patients who do not achieve complete remission are classed as having an event at time zero. A binary outcome measure of being event-free at 8 months post-registration may be assessed to reflect treatment activity on both local and distant disease. This time point corresponds with approximately 3 months after completion of radiotherapy and provides a robust time point at which to assess disease status in the absence of initial post-treatment radiological artefacts. Patients continue to be radiologically assessed every 3 months for the first year after completion of radiotherapy. Therefore this specific time point of interest forms part of the measurement of the overall EFS outcome. These outcome measures, both at 8 months and over the year following completion of radiotherapy, reflect relatively short-term assessments of treatment activity, whereas the primary endpoint of a phase III trial would usually be the longer-term endpoint of OS. Both the binary and overall time-to-event outcome measures are therefore considered as possible primary outcome measures for the phase II trial. The use of a time-to-event endpoint has the potential advantage of providing more information about the pattern of disease recurrence, than simply dichotomising the information at a single time point. However, there are a number of factors contributing to the decision as to which outcome measure to choose as the primary assessment, including available statistical designs, acceptable lengths of follow-up (i.e. follow-up to 8 months only or continued follow-up until event occurrence), randomisation, sample size and design operating characteristic requirements (i.e. type I and II errors).

Randomisation

Drug A is to be given in combination with radiotherapy, that is, another effective treatment modality. It is important that any activity observed with the combination may be attributed to the addition of drug A. Randomisation may, therefore, be incorporated to provide a more robust and reliable assessment of the additional benefit derived from the addition of drug A in this particular setting. Incorporating a formal comparison between the arms will ensure decision-making at the end of phase II is more statistically robust. This is particularly relevant here, since the primary aim of the phase II trial is to make a go/no-go decision regarding proceeding to phase III. While this approach may be more appropriate, at this stage we also consider designs that incorporate randomisation without formally powered statistical comparison to address all possibilities in this setting and allow further discussion with the clinicians.

Design category

It is important that multiple scenarios are considered when choosing the statistical design, to assess how robust each of them is if outcomes in either the experimental or control arm are not as expected. For example, if activity in the control arm is uncertain, how well do the different trial designs cope with an under- or over-estimation of this activity?

Rejected designs:

i. On the basis that proof of concept data for a similar molecularly-targeted agent in combination with radiotherapy already exist, a two-stage or multi-stage approach allowing for early termination for lack of activity was, in this example, deemed unnecessary.

ii. Decision-theoretic approaches to trial design incorporate information on number of patients to be treated in future phase III trials, total number of patients who may benefit from the treatment in the future and costs of treatment. Due to difficulties in reliably determining such information in this situation, a decision-theoretic approach was deemed inappropriate.

iii. Activity with radiotherapy alone is expected to be relatively high in this setting. It is deemed appropriate to only proceed to a phase III trial with drug A if a significant, clinically-relevant improvement in activity is observed, over and above that achieved with radiotherapy alone. A three-outcome design, which allows an 'inconclusive' result to be identified for the primary endpoint, and additional, secondary endpoints to be considered for the purpose of decision-making, was therefore deemed inappropriate for this setting.

iv. Finally, randomised discontinuation designs were also rejected, on the basis that the initial assessment of treatment activity is carried out on completion of treatment. Randomised discontinuation designs are appropriate when it is possible to randomise those patients who are, for example, responding to treatment at a pre-specified, early assessment point, to either continue or discontinue therapy, thus obtaining a randomised comparison of treatment versus no treatment in responders. In this particular trial setting, this opportunity does not arise as patients have only a single block of treatment, so this design is not applicable. It may have been possible to randomise patients who responded to initial radiotherapy to receive or not receive drug A; however, this would not have addressed the central question of whether drug A enhances the activity of radiotherapy.

Candidate designs: One-stage and phase II/III designs were considered as potential designs for the trial.

Possible designs

Thus far, we have determined that the phase II trial will be a randomised study, addressing the go/no-go decision to proceed to a phase III trial, primarily on the basis of activity. This will be assessed on the basis of either a binary outcome measure or a time-to-event outcome measure. Having rejected other potential designs, as in the previous section, the trial will have either a conventional one-stage phase II or phase II/III statistical design. Phase II/III designs allow a relatively seamless transition from phase II to III. They can be more efficient with regard to time, cost and patients, than designing and running separate phase II and III trials. They are also particularly valuable where patient numbers are limited, since it is possible to incorporate data from patients recruited during phase II in the analysis of the phase III trial. However, a potential limitation is that this design precludes incorporating lessons learnt in the phase II trial when designing the subsequent phase III trial.

At this stage, two practical issues are particularly relevant. First, the investigators wish to move rapidly to the phase III trial if there is sufficient evidence of activity. Second, the eligible patient population is very precisely defined, so the available patient population for trial recruitment will be limited. The first point may clearly be a wish of many investigators, but in this particular scenario moving rapidly to phase III may be justified. Previous evidence already exists for the tolerability and efficacy of a similar treatment, albeit in a more advanced disease setting. Therefore, issues surrounding treatment acceptability in the current setting are not expected. Similarly, on the basis of previous evidence in the more advanced setting, there is a high expectation that treatment activity will be observed. In addition, the patient population is well defined and a clear outline of the potential phase III trial protocol is already in place.

The requirement to learn more about the treatment under investigation and the specific target phase III population in order to determine or modify the design of a subsequent phase III trial is therefore minimal. In this respect, it may be deemed feasible to adopt a phase II/III trial design.

Having discussed these considerations in detail, it was ultimately decided that a phase II/III design was most appropriate for the trial in question, with the phase II element designed to have only a single stage.

Phase II/III trials can be designed by incorporating stand-alone phase II designs into a phase III trial, as is the concept described by Storer (1990), and may incorporate different primary outcome measures in each phase. In this respect, stand-alone, one-stage phase II designs may be considered.

Reviewing the one-stage and phase II/III designs in Chapter 4 which fit to a greater or lesser extent the design requirements described above, the following designs may be considered for this trial.

One-stage phase II designs to incorporate into phase II/III:

i. Herson and Carter (1986) – binary outcome, randomisation with no formal comparison between treatment arms

ii. Thall and Simon (1990) – binary outcome, randomisation with no formal comparison between treatment arms

iii. Stone et al. (2007b) and Simon et al. (2001) – time-to-event outcome, randomisation with formal comparison between treatment arms

iv. Chen and Beckman (2009) – time-to-event outcome, randomisation with formal comparison between treatment arms

Phase II/III:

v. Storer (1990) – binary outcome, randomisation with no formal comparison between treatment arms in phase II

vi. Lachin and Younes (2007) – binary or time-to-event outcome, randomisation with formal comparison between treatment arms for lack of activity

vii. Chow and Tu (2008) – binary or time-to-event outcome, randomisation with formal comparison between treatment arms

Stage 3 – Practicalities

Practical considerations for selecting between designs

We now consider each of the above designs in turn.

i and ii. The designs of Herson and Carter and Thall and Simon each incorporate a randomised control arm without the primary intention of formal comparison of this group with the experimental arm. The purpose here is to provide an assessment of the reliability of the results observed in the experimental arm, reducing the influence of bias from factors such as patient selection by having a parallel control arm that puts the experimental arm results into context. With these designs, the decision to proceed to phase III or not is, in theory, based primarily on the results observed in the experimental arm of the trial. The reliability of such a decision, to either claim or refute sufficient activity of the experimental therapy with no formal comparison with the control arm at this stage, may be questioned, especially given the requirement to move seamlessly to phase III on the basis of these results. Additionally, in the design described by Thall and Simon only a proportion of patients are randomised to the control arm, determined to maximise the precision of the estimated experimental treatment effect. In order to incorporate this design into a phase II/III trial, enabling patients recruited during phase II to be incorporated in the phase III analysis, an equal number of patients would be required in each of the control and experimental arms, assuming randomisation on a 1:1 basis in phase III.

iii. Stone and colleagues describe a phase II design which is formally powered to compare the treatment arm with the control arm, using relaxed type I errors and potentially targeting large treatment effects. This reflects the designs described by Simon et al. in the setting of time-to-event outcomes, which are described by the authors as 'phase 2.5 screening' designs, due to the use of phase III-type designs but with type I error rates typically associated with phase II (Simon et al. 2001). By incorporating formal comparison with the control arm, the sample size of the trial will inevitably increase. This should, however, be weighed against the reliability of the decision-making criteria and compared with that for the non-comparative phase II designs described in i and ii above.

iv. Chen and Beckman describe an approach to a randomised phase II trial design that incorporates the ratio of sample sizes between phases II and III. Optimal type I and II errors for the design are identified by means of an efficiency score function. Formal comparison with the control arm is incorporated. The design considers cost efficiency of the phase II and III trials, on the basis of the ratio of sample sizes between phases II and III and the *a priori* probability of success of the investigational treatment. Sufficient detail is provided within the paper to allow implementation and an R program is provided to identify optimal designs.

v. Storer describes the design of a phase II/III trial which corresponds to a single-arm phase II trial design embedded in a randomised phase III trial, such that patients are randomised between control and experimental arms during phase II. However, decision-making is based primarily on the results of the experimental arm. In this respect, the design is similar to those described for i and ii and therefore the same considerations apply here.

vi. The randomised phase II/III design described by Lachin and Younes bases the decision to progress to phase III on an assessment of futility at the end of phase II. Incorporating the expected correlation between the phase II and III outcomes, this design preserves the type I and II errors and enables patients recruited during phase II to be included in the phase III analysis. From a practical viewpoint, this design requires programming to determine sample size and other operating characteristics.

vii. Chow and Tu propose a seamless phase II/III design for scenarios where there is a well-established relationship between the phase II and III endpoints, that is, the phase II endpoint is predictive of the phase III endpoint. This design is based on two separate studies, with differing endpoints and durations, being combined to derive the same objective. As such, data from the phase II trial are used to predict the phase III endpoint, rather than continuing to follow patients, to observe the endpoint. Moreover, in the current trial, we would want to obtain data on both the phase II and phase III primary endpoints in both phases of the trial, requiring longer follow-up of the patients recruited in phase II. For this reason, the design of Chow and Tu is not appropriate for this trial.

Table 8.1 summarises the specific design requirements for the study, as well as the desirable practical elements associated with design selection (relating to software availability in this setting). After further discussion with the clinical team it is agreed that incorporation of a formally powered statistical comparison between the treatment arms is most appropriate in this setting. Bearing this in mind, the two designs that fit the specific study requirements and also have software available to allow easier implementation are (iii) Stone et al. (2007b)/Simon et al. (2001) and (iv) Chen and Beckman (2009). Due to lack of familiarity with the design described by Chen and

Table 8.1   Summary of practical considerations for each design.

Consideration	i	ii	iii	iv	v	vi	vii
Required							
1:1 randomisation	Y	N	Y	Y	Y	Y	Y
Formal comparison with control	N	N	Y	Y	N	Y	Y
Desirable							
Statistical software/programs available	N	N	Y	Y	Y	N	N

Beckman, it was decided that further simulation work to explore this design in more detail would be beneficial. In this particular scenario we may choose the approach described by Stone et al./Simon et al. since this may be immediately implemented. Taking a pragmatic approach to designing this trial, the final proposed statistical design is a randomised phase II design following Stone et al. (2007b), embedded in a phase III trial.

Proposed trial design

Giving further consideration to the primary endpoint of the phase II trial, it is important to highlight that the intention of this study is ultimately to run seamlessly into a phase III trial. Any patients entered into the phase II trial would, therefore, have exactly the same eligibility criteria and be followed up in exactly the same manner as patients entered in the phase III element, that is, patient follow-up within the trial would *not* cease once the initial 8-month endpoint, described earlier, had been observed. In this sense, the phase II trial accrues further data on overall EFS beyond the 8-month time point. Since this overall time-to-event endpoint has been shown to be correlated with OS in locally-advanced HNSCC, it seems prudent to incorporate as much information on this endpoint as possible in phase II, rather than dichotomising the information at a single time point and consequently ignoring data beyond this. We therefore chose to use time-to-event EFS as the primary endpoint for the phase II trial, with a specific evaluation of 8-month EFS as a secondary endpoint.

On the basis of previously published EFS data in a similar patient population, the expected median EFS with radiotherapy alone is 1 year (Tobias et al. 2010). In the more advanced setting, a reduction in hazard rate for EFS of 30% (95% CI 0.54–0.90) was observed with the addition of a similar molecularly-targeted agent to radiotherapy alone, corresponding to a 27% reduction in hazard rate for OS. In order to observe a slightly larger treatment effect in the current population, a reduction in hazard rate for EFS of approximately 35% with the addition of drug A to radiotherapy is targeted, corresponding to an improved median EFS of 6.5 months (from 12 to 18.5 months). Assuming patients are recruited over a 2-year period, with all patients being followed up for a minimum of 8 months, our chosen design would require 84 patients per arm (with 96 events overall) to detect a hazard ratio of 0.65 with 80% power and a one-sided 10% significance level (i.e. there is a 10% chance that we would declare the addition of drug A to radiotherapy superior to radiotherapy alone on the basis of EFS, and thus continue into the phase III trial, when in fact there is no difference).

The corresponding phase III component of the trial is designed to detect an improvement in hazard rate for OS of 25%, that is, HR 0.75. Although there is correlation between the phase II and III primary outcome measures, the correlation between the treatment effects observed in each phase is not expected to be perfect. Thus we would expect a smaller treatment effect on OS than on EFS. Median OS with radiotherapy alone is expected to be approximately 2.6 years on the basis of previously published data in a similar patient population (Tobias et al. 2010). With 80% power

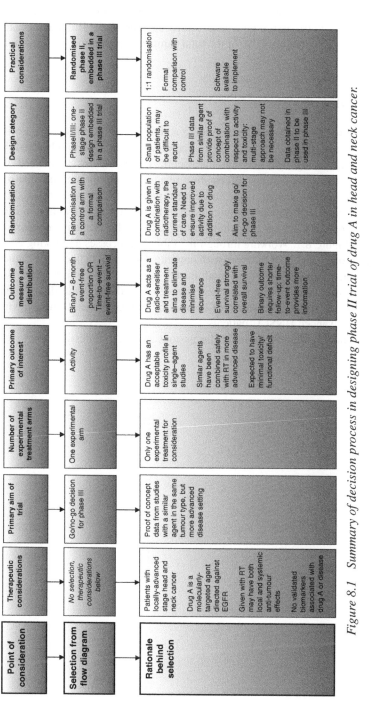

Figure 8.1 Summary of decision process in designing phase II trial of drug A in head and neck cancer.

and a 5% two-sided significance level, 283 patients per arm are required (with 382 deaths overall), assuming 5-year follow-up. The phase II component therefore comprises approximately 30% of the total sample size required for the whole phase II/III trial.

Summary

This trial has been designed to assess the activity of the addition of a molecularly-targeted cytostatic agent, drug A, to radiotherapy in locally-advanced HNSCC patients. By taking into account therapeutic considerations associated with the drug, the patient population, information regarding appropriate outcome measures in HNSCC and the design of the subsequent phase III trial, we addressed the trial-specific design requirements through each of the three stages featured in Figure 2.1 and described in Chapter 2. A summary of each of the elements addressed is presented in Figure 8.1. Working through the thought processes and taking an iterative approach to the design of the trial, with ongoing discussion between the clinician and statistician, we have designed a randomised, controlled, seamless phase II/III trial which incorporates formal comparison between radiotherapy plus drug A and radiotherapy alone, for the assessment of EFS as the primary phase II outcome measure, in locally-advanced HNSCC patients.

We thank Dr Mehmet Senn for discussions around trial design.

9

Combination chemotherapy in second-line treatment of non-small cell lung cancer

Ornella Belvedere and Sarah Brown

Established treatment options for patients with advanced-stage non-small cell lung cancer (NSCLC) previously treated with chemotherapy include single-agent chemotherapy (i.e. docetaxel in unselected patients or pemetrexed in patients with nonsquamous histology) and oral tyrosine kinase inhibitors (i.e. erlotinib or gefitinib) (Azzoli et al. 2009). The use of doublet chemotherapy is currently being investigated using various chemotherapy combinations. Drug B is a cytotoxic with a favourable toxicity profile and evidence of activity in combination with docetaxel in the first-line setting for NSCLC patients. To date, drug B has not been investigated in second-line combination therapy. It is hypothesised that drug B, in combination with docetaxel, will improve the efficacy of docetaxel alone for patients with advanced-stage NSCLC. The trial is proposed to run as an academic study in a small number of centres with limited funding and relatively few patients; historical control data in this population are, however, available. A phase II trial of drug B in combination with docetaxel is proposed to determine whether a larger phase III trial should be planned and considered for funding by a much larger collaborative group.

A Practical Guide to Designing Phase II Trials in Oncology, First Edition.
Sarah R. Brown, Walter M. Gregory, Chris Twelves and Julia Brown.
© 2014 John Wiley & Sons, Ltd. Published 2014 by John Wiley & Sons, Ltd.

Stage 1 – Trial questions

Therapeutic considerations

Mechanism of action: Drug B is a platinum-based cytotoxic agent expected to induce tumour response. It has a lack of cross-resistance with other platinum-based agents used in first-line NSCLC, based on pre-clinical data. Its favourable toxicity profile, along with evidence of activity in NSCLC in both pre-clinical and clinical studies (Monnet et al. 1998), makes drug B a good candidate to combine with docetaxel in NSCLC.

Aim of treatment: The ultimate goal of second-line therapy for NSCLC is to prolong patients' survival. Additionally, controlling disease-related symptoms and improving quality of life are important in this setting. An appropriate early indicator of treatment activity for combination chemotherapy which is expected to induce cell kill is achieving radiological tumour response.

Single or combination therapy: Drug B is to be given in combination with docetaxel, an active drug, therefore any activity of the combination therapy would need to be shown as over and above that of docetaxel alone.

Biomarkers: There are no validated biomarkers associated with drug B or with NSCLC, to allow patient enrichment or alternative assessment of therapeutic activity.

Primary intention of trial

Proof of concept data are available for this combination as first-line treatment for NSCLC. A proof of concept study for drug B in combination with docetaxel is, therefore, not deemed necessary. The aim of the current trial is to determine the activity of drug B in combination with docetaxel in patients with NSCLC previously treated with chemotherapy, to make a go/no-go decision as to whether or not to proceed to a phase III trial.

Number of experimental treatment arms

There is only one experimental treatment under investigation therefore a selection trial is not required.

Primary outcome of interest

Drug B has an acceptable toxicity profile in single-agent studies and has a mild toxicity profile in combination with docetaxel when assessed in chemo-naïve patients. Therefore, while toxicity will form a secondary endpoint of the phase II trial, the primary outcome of interest is activity alone.

Stage 2 – Design components

Outcome measure and distribution

The primary aim of treatment in patients with advanced NSCLC previously treated with chemotherapy is ultimately to prolong overall survival. Early indicators of treatment activity are radiological tumour response, since the cytotoxic combination treatment under investigation is expected to induce tumour cell kill, and progression-free survival (PFS). The strength of the relationship between response rate, PFS and overall survival in NSCLC has been investigated in patients with advanced NSCLC (Mandrekar et al. 2010). PFS was shown to be more strongly correlated with overall survival than response; however, the analysis is based on a limited number of trials, some of which incorporate targeted therapies that may be expected to induce tumour stabilisation rather than response. Since the focus of the current study is on cytotoxic treatment, it was deemed appropriate to assess response rate as the primary outcome measure. Thus, a binary outcome measure of the proportion of patients achieving at least a confirmed partial response will be used.

Randomisation

Drug B is to be given in combination with docetaxel. It is important to be confident that any apparent extra activity with the combination can reasonably be attributed to the addition of drug B. Randomisation should, therefore, be incorporated to provide robust and reliable results in this particular setting. Incorporating formal statistical comparison between the arms provides the most robust approach; however, as acknowledged in Chapter 2, this requires a major increase in sample size compared to single-arm phase II trials, unless a large treatment effect is targeted. Here, with the trial proposed to run in a small number of centres and with relatively few patients, formally powered comparison with single agent docetaxel may be prohibitive in terms of sample size. There is a substantial body of historical data available on the activity of docetaxel alone in second-line NSCLC, which can reliably inform the expected response rate (Fossella et al. 2000; Hanna et al. 2004; Shepherd et al. 2000). It may, however, be plausible to incorporate randomisation but with no formally powered comparison in this trial. As discussed in Chapter 2, without formal comparison between the control and experimental arm, the sample size increase is more modest than when a formal comparison is intended. In its simplest form, the sample size may just be doubled, to allocate patients in a 1:1 ratio to control and experimental treatments. Here the control arm acts as a calibration group, and the inclusion of randomisation reduces patient selection bias, thus providing greater confidence interpreting results of the experimental therapy.

Design category

It is important that multiple scenarios be considered when choosing the statistical design, to assess how robust each of them is, if outcomes in either the experimental or control arm are not as expected. For example, if activity in the control arm is uncertain, how well do the different trial designs cope with an under- or over-estimation of this activity?

Rejected designs:

i. Proof of concept data for the combination of drug B with docetaxel are available in the first-line NSCLC setting. There is no reason to expect that the combination will be less active than docetaxel alone; the safety profile of the combination is known and will be monitored throughout the trial. On this basis, two-stage, multi-stage and continuous monitoring approaches allowing for early termination for lack of activity are not necessary.

ii. Decision-theoretic approaches to trial design incorporate information on number of patients to be treated in future phase III trials, total number of patients who may benefit from the treatment in the future and costs of treatment. Due to difficulties in reliably determining such data in this particular setting, a decision-theoretic approach was deemed inappropriate.

iii. Randomised discontinuation designs were also rejected. In the context of combination chemotherapy for NSCLC a randomised discontinuation design might mean all patients initially receiving drug B and docetaxel, and those who respond then being randomised to continue or stop drug B. Such a design would not, however, truly evaluate the combination versus single-agent question, as all participants would have received drug B and docetaxel.

iv. Finally, since the resources to run a phase III trial are not available and would be contingent on the results of this study, the trial is intended as a stand-alone phase II trial. Phase II/III designs may therefore also be discarded.

Candidate designs: One-stage and three-outcome designs were considered as potential designs for the trial.

Possible designs

We have determined that the phase II trial will be a randomised trial, addressing the go/no-go decision to proceed to a phase III trial, principally on the basis of activity. This will be assessed using a binary outcome measure via either a one-stage or three-outcome statistical design. It is expected that formal comparison between docetaxel and docetaxel + drug B would result in a prohibitive sample size; nevertheless, these designs are considered in order to explore the possibility of incorporating this. In order to also consider randomisation with no formal comparison, that is, where the control arm acts as calibration, single-arm trial designs are included with decision-making criteria based primarily on the results of the experimental arm alone. Reviewing the available designs in Chapters 3 and 4 which fit these design parameters, the following designs may to a greater or lesser extent be appropriate. Discussion as to selecting between these specific designs is given in the next section.

One-stage:

From Chapter 3:

   i. Fleming (1982) – single-arm design

  ii. Fazzari et al. (2000) – single-arm design

 iii. A'Hern (2001) – single-arm design

 iv. Chang et al. (2004) – single-arm design

  v. Mayo and Gajewski (2004) – single-arm design

 vi. Gajewski and Mayo (2006) – single-arm design

vii. Vickers (2009) – single-arm design

From Chapter 4:

viii. Herson and Carter (1986) – randomisation with no formal comparison between treatment arms

 ix. Thall and Simon (1990) – randomisation with no formal comparison between treatment arms

  x. Stone et al. (2007b) – randomisation with formal comparison between treatment arms

Three outcomes:

From Chapter 3:

 xi. Storer (1992) – single-arm design

xii. Sargent et al. (2001) – single-arm design

From Chapter 4:

xiii. Hong and Wang (2007) – randomisation with formal comparison between treatment arms

Stage 3 – Practicalities

Practical considerations for selecting between designs

The three-outcome designs listed above may be seen as sub-designs of a one-stage design and may be used when there is a region of uncertainty between, for example, the response rate that clearly warrants further investigation in phase III and one that definitely does not. If the primary outcome measure of a three-outcome design trial is inconclusive, the decision to move to phase III or not may be based on other factors, such as safety or cost. Three-outcome designs may also require fewer patients than some two-outcome designs using the same design criteria. In order to assess potential savings in patient numbers and the impact on operating characteristics associated with this, we consider below each of the one-stage and three-outcome designs relevant to the proposed trial.

i. Fleming outlines a single-stage design based on rejecting the null hypothesis that the response rate is less than or equal to a pre-specified value, typically that associated with the current control arm. Sample size calculation assumes the normal approximation to the binomial distribution; therefore, where small sample sizes are identified the robustness of this assumption may be questionable. Software is readily available to implement this design.

ii. Fazzari et al. describe the design of a phase II trial based on estimating the phase III outcome measure parameter and corresponding $x\%$ confidence interval, with decision criteria based around the upper bound of the confidence interval. The authors describe the design as an 'intermediate trial between a screening phase II manuscript and the phase III randomised comparative survival manuscript' (Fazzari et al. 2000). This design is not appropriate to the current setting since the ability to reliably predict the phase III endpoint of overall survival based on response is questionable. The design requires programming to allow implementation.

iii. The design of A'Hern is an adaptation of the Fleming design described above. Here the sample size and decision criteria are based on the exact binomial distribution and may therefore be more appropriate for small sample sizes. Software is readily available to implement this design.

iv. Chang et al. propose a single-arm design that incorporates the number of patients on which the historical control data are based. The design focuses on performing an exact unconditional test comparing the observed historical control event rate with the expected event rate in the experimental arm. The authors note that in many cases the sample sizes determined were similar to those derived under alternative single-arm non-comparative designs. Programs are noted as being available from the authors.

v. Mayo and Gajewski propose a Bayesian single-arm design based on the use of informative priors, either pessimistic or optimistic. Various approaches to sample size calculation are detailed based on the mean, median or mode prior. It is noted that these different approaches can result in very different trial designs, which is largely due to the method of eliciting the prior information and its interpretation. In the current setting where there are reliable historical control data on single-agent docetaxel, and results using the combination, albeit in a different clinical setting, this design may not be necessary or appropriate. The design requires programming to allow implementation.

vi. The second design of Gajewski and Mayo is based on the use of conflicting prior information, whereby both pessimistic *and* optimistic assumptions are incorporated. Sample size is determined via an iterative approach and therefore requires some programming. As with the previous design, given the available data in the current setting, the decision was taken to consider more appropriate alternative designs. The design requires programming to allow implementation.

vii. The design of Vickers uses historical control data to generate a statistical prediction model to predict the results of the experimental arm in the current trial. The observed results at the end of the trial are then compared with this prediction. Where the historical control cohort is of a sufficiently large size, the resulting trial design using this methodology will require a similar number of patients to a single-arm trial designed on the basis of comparison of proportions. Given the historical control data available in the current setting are sufficiently large, and the additional complexities associated with building a prediction model for the proposed design, a practical decision was made not to consider this design. Stata programs are provided in the appendix to the manuscript.

viii. Herson and Carter incorporate a randomised control arm without formal comparison of this group with the experimental arm. The purpose here is to provide an assessment of the reliability of the results observed in the experimental arm and also to assess in detail the activity of the control arm. This allows evaluation of the assumptions made in designing the trial and provides additional information particularly in the event of rejecting the alternative hypothesis of increased activity in the control arm. The overall design is a combination of individual designs for each of the control and experimental arms and may result in overall sample sizes of between three and five times that of a non-calibrated design. This relatively large increase in sample size is inefficient in the current setting where there is a body of historical control data available. From a practical viewpoint, this design may also require programming to determine sample size if operating characteristics do not equal those provided in the manuscript.

ix. In the design of Thall and Simon fewer patients are randomised to the control arm than to the experimental arm to maximise the precision of the response rate in the experimental arm relative to the control. The proportion randomised to the control arm is dependent upon the amount of historical control data, the degree of variability and the overall sample size of the phase II study being planned (calculated using formulae provided). From a practical viewpoint, this design requires programming to determine sample size and other operating characteristics iteratively.

x. Stone and colleagues describe a phase II design which is formally powered to compare the experimental arm with the control arm, using relaxed type I errors and targeting large treatment effects, using typical designs considered for phase III. This design will, therefore, result in larger sample sizes than others. Software is readily available to implement this design.

Three outcomes:

xi. Storer proposes a three-outcome design adapted from a typical single-stage design. Here, if the observed event rate is between that specified under the null hypothesis ($p1$) and that specified under the alternative ($p2$), it is possible to consider additional information before deciding either in favour of or against the experimental arm. The event rate of uncertainty is taken to be around $(p1 + p2)/2$. The error associated with incorrectly concluding in favour of either the null or alternative hypotheses is specified under this event rate. Software is not available for this method and would therefore require programming; a table of various design scenarios is, however, given.

xii. Sargent et al. describe a three-outcome design similar to that described by Storer. Here the errors associated with incorrectly declaring an inconclusive result under the null and under the alternative hypotheses are specified and are allowed to differ. This allows more flexibility in the design of the trial. With the addition of a region of uncertainty, sample sizes are typically less than those derived under a two-outcome design with the same operating characteristics. A table of various design scenarios is given; programs may be available from the authors upon request.

xiii. Hong and Wang describe a randomised three-outcome design whereby decision-making is based on the difference in the number of events observed between the arms, with the null hypothesis that there is no difference. The design incorporates formal comparison with the control arm. The region of uncertainty for this three-outcome design falls around the middle region between the null and alternative hypothesis (that the difference is at least Δ). Software is noted as being available upon request from the authors to enable the operating characteristics to be identified; we were, however, unable to obtain this.

The key practical consideration in deciding between the designs described above is the ability to implement the methodology to enable a comparison of sample sizes and operating characteristics between the designs. Table 9.1 summarises the desirable practical elements associated with design selection (relating to software availability in this setting) and the additional considerations made in each of the summaries above. The six designs that were therefore considered, that is, those with no additional methodological complexities for this scenario and where software is available, are (i) Fleming, (iii) A'Hern, (iv) Chang et al., (x) Stone et al. and (xii) Sargent et al.

Proposed trial design

The expected response rate with docetaxel alone in this setting is 7–10% (Fossella et al. 2000; Hanna et al. 2004; Shepherd et al. 2000). To decide whether or not to further investigate the activity of docetaxel + drug B in the phase III setting, a response rate below which further investigation would not be warranted was set at 10%. The targeted response rate of docetaxel + drug B was set at 30%, chosen as being the minimal clinically-relevant response rate that would warrant further investigation of this combination therapy, that is, a 20% absolute increase in response rate.

To consider each of the possible designs, the following operating characteristics were defined. For the one-stage two-outcome designs, a one-sided type I error rate of

Table 9.1 Summary of practical considerations for each design.

Consideration			Design			
	i	ii	iii	iv	v	vi	vii
Additional complexities in methodological approach?	N	Y	N	N	Y	Y	Y
Statistical software/ programs available	Y	N	Y	Y	N	N	Y
Other information	–	Based on phase III primary outcome	–	Formal comparison with historical control data	–	–	–

Consideration			Design			
	viii	ix	x	xi	xii	xiii
Additional complexities in methodological approach?	N	N	N	N	N	N
Statistical software/ programs available	N	N	Y	N	Y	N^a
Other information	Imbalanced randomisation in favour of control	–	Incorporates formal comparison	–	–	Incorporates formal comparison

[a]Noted as being available upon request; however, we were unable to obtain.

5% and 80% power are used. For the three-outcome design, a one-sided type I error rate, α, of 5% and 80% power (i.e. the probability of rejecting the null hypothesis when the alternative is true) are again used; however, additional error rates of incorrectly declaring an inconclusive result also require specifying (see Section 2.2.3.6 for full details). The probability of incorrectly declaring an inconclusive result when in fact the alternative hypothesis is true, δ (i.e. response rate $\geq 30\%$), and the probability of incorrectly declaring an inconclusive result when in fact the null hypothesis is true, λ (i.e. response rate $\leq 10\%$), may be specified separately. In the current example we take $\delta = 10\%$ and $\lambda = 15\%$. To maintain 80% power under the three-outcome design, the probability of incorrectly rejecting the alternative hypothesis when in fact it is true, β, is set to 10%.

Table 9.2 summarises the required sample sizes and associated stopping criteria for the operating characteristics described earlier. The design based on Chang et al. is taken from the published sample size tables, assuming historical control data available for a minimum of 120 patients; it is acknowledged that there is in fact a much larger body of data available for this population.

Considering each of the designs, that of Sargent et al. was chosen, including randomisation to a control arm to guard against selection bias and provide a calibration arm. The randomised design incorporating formal comparison (Stone et al. 2007b) requires approximately twice the number of patients per arm compared to those where no formal comparison is intended. Due to the prohibitive sample size of this design for few study centres, this was not used. The sample sizes for the one-stage designs of Fleming and A'Hern are comparable to that of the three-outcome design. Although the design of Fleming requires one less patient per arm, the inclusion of the

Table 9.2   Summary of sample sizes and stopping rules under each design.

Design	N (per arm)	Stopping criteria
Stone et al.	49	Formal comparison; based on one-sided p-value $< 5\%$
Fleming	20	If at least 5/20 responses observed, further investigation warranted
A'Hern	25	If at least 6/25 responses observed, further investigation warranted
Chang et al.	29	Exact unconditional test of observed response rate compared to historical control data
Sargent et al.	21	If number of responses observed in experimental arm (r) is • ≤ 3 – no further investigation warranted • ≥ 5 – further investigation warranted • $3 < r < 5$ – inconclusive – consider alternative outcomes

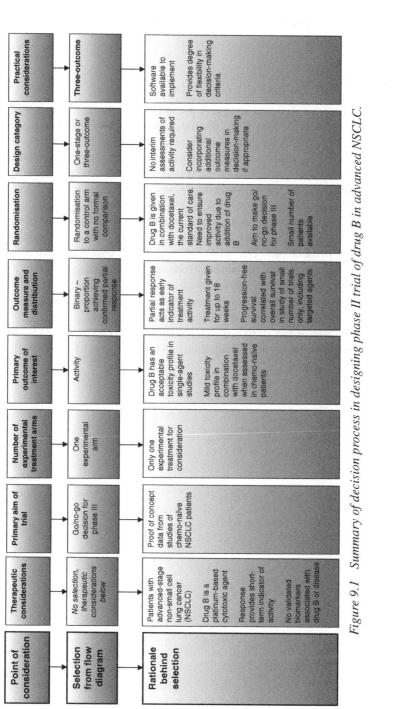

Figure 9.1 Summary of decision process in designing phase II trial of drug B in advanced NSCLC.

inconclusive region with just one additional patient per arm provides extra flexibility in this situation.

Summary

This trial has been designed to assess the activity of the addition of a platinum-based cytotoxic agent, drug B, to docetaxel as second-line treatment for patients with advanced NSCLC. By taking into account the therapeutic considerations associated with the drug, the patient population, literature regarding appropriate outcome measures in NSCLC and methodological issues associated with relevant statistical designs, we addressed the trial-specific design requirements and practical considerations listed in each of the three stages featured in Figure 2.1 and described in Chapter 2. A summary of the discussions associated with each of the eight elements is presented in Figure 9.1. Working through the thought process and taking an iterative approach to the design of the trial, with ongoing discussion between the clinician and statistician, a randomised, controlled, one-stage, three-outcome trial of docetaxel plus drug B for second-line treatment of advanced NSCLC patients was chosen, with response rate as the phase II primary outcome measure, incorporating randomisation to a control arm of single-agent docetaxel for calibration only.

This trial was in fact designed, conducted, analysed and reported by the Alpe-Adria Thoracic Oncology Multidisciplinary (ATOM) group (ATOM019) (Belvedere et al. 2011).

10

Selection by biomarker in prostate cancer

Rick Kaplan and Sarah Brown

There is currently no standard treatment for patients with biochemical-failure-only prostate cancer following curative intent local therapy, the standard of care being watchful waiting. Clinicians are, however, increasingly treating such patients with androgen-deprivation therapies. These have an associated toxicity profile, and there is no conclusive prospective evidence of clinical benefit in this setting. There is, therefore, a need to investigate novel strategies in these patients; immune-modulator strategies may offer an alternative and less-toxic approach for patients with low tumour burden. Vaccine C is a targeted active immunotherapy, hypothesised to control tumour growth (indirectly reflected by prostate specific antigen (PSA) levels) thus potentially prolonging disease-free survival or, at a minimum, postponing exposure to long-term androgen deprivation. The development pathway of treatments in prostate cancer is important to consider in the design of clinical trials. In the setting of biochemical-failure-only prostate cancer, the time from entering clinical development to registration of successful treatments can be particularly long. Phase III trials in this setting may use endpoints such as time to failure of hormone therapy, or time to development of metastatic disease, as surrogates for overall survival. Even so, such events may be uncommon and are delayed often by many years; Pound et al. found that in some settings the median time to development of metastatic disease in untreated men with rising PSA was 8 years (Pound et al. 1999). Thus, consideration of the whole development pathway from phase I to registration is critical to ensure the design of the most efficient clinical trials. In this setting, and example, consideration

A Practical Guide to Designing Phase II Trials in Oncology, First Edition.
Sarah R. Brown, Walter M. Gregory, Chris Twelves and Julia Brown.
© 2014 John Wiley & Sons, Ltd. Published 2014 by John Wiley & Sons, Ltd.

is given to expanding the phase II trial immediately to phase III, should the vaccine be shown to be associated with an encouraging level of activity.

Stage 1 – Trial questions

Therapeutic considerations

Mechanism of action: Vaccine C is a targeted active immunotherapy. It induces MUC1 antigen expression to induce both innate and adaptive immunity. The vaccine is likely to be of interest for patients with low-volume tumours or patients with biochemical failure only, since although these patients have other treatment options available to them, they do not necessarily need them at this time. In addition, vaccines are generally expected to be more effective when tumour volume is minimal.

Aim of treatment: The ultimate aim of treatment of patients with biochemical-failure-only disease is reversal of rising levels of PSAs, so as to delay onset of disease, delay of complications and improvement in metastatic disease-free survival.

Single or combination therapy: Vaccine C is given as a single agent.

Biomarkers: In this population of patients, the biomarker PSA is an appropriate intermediate outcome measure of disease activity (see Section 10.2.1 for further discussion). There are no biomarkers associated with potential for benefit from vaccine C for the purpose of population enrichment.

Primary intention of trial

The overall aims of the trial are to first identify an encouraging signal with vaccine C to warrant further study and then to select a single dosing schedule to investigate further in a randomised phase III trial. Proof of concept data are available for this vaccine in non-small cell lung cancer, but not in prostate cancer, although studies of similar agents have been performed. The trial aims to provide proof of concept data in this setting as well as sufficient evidence of activity to make a go/no-go decision as to whether or not to proceed to a phase III trial and to select the most active dose of vaccine C to compare against watchful waiting in the phase III trial.

Number of experimental treatment arms

Two dosing schedules are to be considered: (1) weekly to week 7 then every 3 weeks to week 36 or progressive disease (PD); (2) every 3 weeks to week 36 or PD. The intention is not to show that one schedule is superior to the other, but to guide selection so that the selected schedule is sufficiently active to warrant investigation in a randomised controlled phase III trial.

Primary outcome of interest

Safety and tolerability of the vaccine have been established in phase I trials, and there have been previous phase II studies of the vaccine in non-small cell lung cancer. Toxicity assessment is not thought appropriate as a primary outcome measure, since previous studies suggest this vaccine is less toxic than alternatives such as androgen-deprivation therapy; toxicity will therefore form a secondary endpoint, with the primary endpoint activity alone. Since the current standard of treatment for these patients is watchful waiting, and these patients are asymptomatic, a substantial improvement in activity is needed to warrant further investigation in a phase III trial. The primary outcome of interest is therefore activity alone.

Stage 2 – Design components

Outcome measure and distribution

There are several outcome measures in trials of targeted therapies in prostate cancer (Stadler 2002). In this group of patients tumour burden is low and patients are asymptomatic. These patients have biochemical-failure-only disease that often predates clinical progression by a considerable time; therefore, endpoints such as time to development of metastatic disease are impractical due to the long follow-up times required. PSA is a commonly used short-term biomarker of outcome in prostate cancer and may be an appropriate primary outcome in this setting. Although PSA has not been shown to be a true surrogate for overall survival in the context of predicting treatment effects, a strong correlation between PSA and overall survival has been shown for the individual patient (Collette et al. 2005). A correlation was, however, also shown for PSA response. PSA response has previously been used in phase II trials, as an endpoint to determine when *not* to take a treatment forward for further investigation, since if a patient does not achieve a PSA response, he is unlikely to gain any further clinical benefit from treatment. Using PSA response as a robust outcome to reliably suggest further evaluation in phase III is warranted may, however, be questioned. The use of PSA response relies on pre-defined definitions which may not reflect the longitudinal trajectory of PSA levels over time. By assessing PSA as a continuous variable, and comparing changes over time, we may obtain more information on the effect of treatment than we would by using a simple binary outcome of PSA response. The use of PSA doubling time (PSA DT), derived from changes in PSA over time, is a commonly referenced outcome measure that is significantly associated with risk of prostate cancer-specific mortality (Freedland et al. 2005). PSA DT is defined as the natural log of 2 (0.693) divided by the estimate of the slope of the regression line of log(PSA) over time. PSA DT data are more widely published than change in PSA levels at a specific time point and provide an appropriate short-term measure of the activity of the vaccine that does not rely on pre-defined response definitions. We assess the pattern of change in PSA levels over time, with the expectation that the use of vaccine C will increase the doubling time. Thus the outcome under consideration is a continuous measure.

Randomisation

Vaccine C is given as a single agent. The current standard of care in this setting is watchful waiting. With the additional complexities associated with giving patients a treatment, such as possible side effects, additional hospital attendances, additional clinical tests and so on, it is important that any treatment effect observed is substantial, to justify the associated 'medicalisation'. The primary outcome measure is PSA DT. PSA levels are expected to rise in patients undergoing watchful waiting, and with the use of vaccine C the rate of rise in PSA is expected to be reduced or even reversed, and therefore PSA DT extended. Inclusion of a control arm is therefore essential to allow comparable data regarding the trajectory of PSA levels over time, which may be dependent upon baseline PSA levels and/or the variable natural history of prostate cancers. It is, however, unlikely that a treatment would be taken forward to phase III if it did not induce initial reductions in PSA levels; therefore, this may also be required by the study sponsor.

There is a wide clinical range of behaviours for biochemical tumours, even more so in prostate cancer than in other cancers. It is important to minimise the chance of random selection of a cohort of patients with a particularly indolent biochemical tumour which may not be applicable to the general disease population. The inclusion of randomisation to a control arm of watchful waiting helps guard against this bias. As previously highlighted, consideration is given to a phase II/III design to speed up the drug development pathway in a setting where clinical events are delayed. In order for such a design to be possible, whereby patients recruited to the phase II element are also then included in the phase III component, it is essential that the control arm of the phase III trial be incorporated from the beginning of the trial, that is, it is an essential design criteria that randomisation is included in the phase II trial. Inclusion of a control arm also allows direct comparison with each of the dosing schedules during the phase II element thus providing a robust assessment of the decision as to whether or not to proceed to phase III. This also follows the discussion of Stadler regarding phase II trial design for trials of cytostatic treatments in prostate cancer (Stadler 2002). Randomisation with formal comparison will, therefore, be incorporated.

Design category

Rejected designs:

i. Currently there are only phase I data with this vaccine in this setting, although phase II studies in non-small cell lung cancer have demonstrated its activity. A two-stage, or multi-stage, design incorporates interim assessments of the activity of the vaccine and can allow early termination for lack of activity, or early selection of a dosing schedule, as well as assessment of safety and tolerability. These designs may, therefore, be deemed appropriate due to the limited experience with this vaccine to date and may allow early dose selection. However, due to inherent logistical problems with multi-stage designs, especially the long follow-up period required before the primary outcome measure is observed (relative to patient recruitment), designs with more than two stages are not considered for this trial.

ii. Likewise, continuous monitoring designs are also not considered.

iii. Since an interim assessment of activity is deemed useful in this setting, the use of one-stage designs was also rejected.

iv. Decision-theoretic approaches to trial design incorporate information on number of patients to be treated in future phase III trials, total patient horizon and costs of treatment. Due to difficulties in reliably determining such information, especially where the underlying disease has a relatively long natural history, a decision-theoretic approach was not considered.

v. The overall aims of the trial are to first identify an encouraging signal with vaccine C to warrant further study and then to select a single dosing schedule to investigate further in a randomised phase III trial. As previously discussed, a substantial treatment effect must be observed compared to watchful waiting alone, to warrant further study. On this basis, the three-outcome design may not be suitable given this incorporates the possibility of an inconclusive result.

vi. Finally, randomised discontinuation designs were also rejected. They do not lend themselves to dose selection studies, and given the consideration for the trial to be expanded into a phase III trial, the use of a concurrent observation control arm is necessary. This design was therefore not considered on this basis.

Candidate designs: Two-stage and phase II/III designs were considered as potential designs for the trial.

Possible designs

Thus far, we have determined that the phase II trial will be a randomised dose selection study, addressing the go/no-go decision to proceed to a phase III trial with a selected schedule of vaccine C, on the basis of activity. This will be assessed using the tumour marker PSA as a continuous outcome measure to derive PSA DT, with the aim of taking forward a single dose to phase III. The use of a phase II/III trial design is of particular interest in this setting due to their associated efficiencies. Phase II/III designs allow a relatively seamless transition from phase II to phase III. They can be more efficient with regard to time, cost and patients, than designing and running separate phase II and III trials. They are particularly efficient where patient numbers are limited or where the time taken to observe phase III events is particularly long, since it is possible to incorporate data from patients recruited during phase II in the analysis of the phase III trial. These considerations are relevant for the current study.

A relevant issue when considering the use of a phase II/III design is that this may preclude the opportunity to learn between trial phases. The chance to reflect on the design of the phase II trial, for example, assessing the impact of issues such as eligibility criteria, can be important when there may be uncertainties around the design of the subsequent phase III trial. In this particular setting, the practical issues associated with moving to phase III as quickly and efficiently as possible, and the ability to include phase II patients with long follow-up times in the phase III component, outweigh the potential benefits of pausing between phases. At the end of the phase II component, recruitment may continue until the phase II analysis is complete. At this time, should the decision to continue into phase III be confirmed, a full review of the phase II component may be conducted to allow any necessary amendments to the trial protocol.

As previously discussed, the use of a two-stage design allows an interim assessment of activity, enabling the possibility to terminate the trial early for either activity or lack of activity or enabling early dose selection. Early termination on the basis that vaccine C is active is not appropriate as the aim is to choose between two potentially active schedules. Early dose selection or termination for lack of activity may, however, be useful.

Phase II/III trials can be designed by incorporating stand-alone phase II designs into a phase III trial, described by Storer (1990), and may incorporate different primary outcome measures in each phase. Stand-alone two-stage phase II selection designs may therefore be included when considering phase II/III trials.

It is possible to conduct selection trials that are designed with go/no-go decision criteria applied to each individual arm separately, after which only those arms deemed sufficiently active (i.e. passing the 'go' criteria) are compared for selection. Such an approach is described by Simon et al. (1985) in the context of binary outcomes. However, in order to minimise the number of designs to be considered and discussed in this specific example, this approach will not be considered here. In practice, such designs may be investigated further.

Reviewing the available two-stage and phase II/III treatment selection designs in Chapter 5 which fit the design parameters described above, the following designs may be considered for this trial.

Two-stage phase II designs to incorporate into phase II/III:

　　i. Levy et al. (2006) – continuous outcome, randomisation with formal comparison with control

　　ii. Shun et al. (2008) – continuous outcome, randomisation with formal comparison with control

Phase II/III (different primary outcome measures at phase II and phase III):

　　iii. Todd and Stallard (2005) – continuous outcome, randomisation with formal comparison with control

　　iv. Liu and Pledger (2005) – continuous outcome, randomisation with formal comparison with control

　　v. Shun et al. (2008) – continuous outcome, randomisation with formal comparison with control

Stage 3 – Practicalities

Practical considerations for selecting between designs

We now consider each of the above designs in turn.

i. The design of Levy et al. incorporates the ability to select a dosing regimen at the end of the first stage of the trial. Treatment selection is based on informal comparison of the two dosing regimens, with no comparison to the control for treatment selection. The treatment with the 'best' outcome (e.g. longest mean PSA DT) is selected as the one to be taken forward for further study. The sample size for the trial is calculated to ensure that the probability that the better treatment is selected is at least 80%, when the true difference between the treatments is a least δ, a pre-specified minimal change. A futility analysis is incorporated to compare the selected treatment with control. The design requires programming as standard programs are not noted as being available.

ii. The design described by Shun et al. incorporates treatment selection at the end of the first stage, where the treatment with the 'better' outcome is selected, and formal superiority comparison with the control at the end of the second stage, conditional on the interim selection. No early termination for lack of activity is proposed at the end of the first stage. The probability of correctly selecting the treatment with the most activity can be pre-specified in the design, as can the timing of the first-stage analysis. The design requires programming.

iii. Todd and Stallard describe a phase II/III design incorporating schedule selection at the end of phase II, which is conducted as a one-stage design. At the end of phase II formal comparisons are made with the control arm and the most superior schedule is selected; termination of the trial at this stage is permitted only for lack of activity. Phase III is then conducted in a group-sequential approach. Programs to calculate stopping boundaries are noted as being available from the authors.

iv. Liu and Pledger propose a phase II/III design which assumes both the phase II and III outcomes are continuous. Treatment selection occurs at the end of phase II, which is conducted in a single stage. At this point, more than one treatment can be selected, and adjustment of the phase III sample size is possible. The design is described in the context of dose selection, whereby at the end of phase II doses with unacceptable toxicity or low activity are dropped. The design requires programming.

v. The design described by Shun et al. in the context of the phase II/III setting is the same as that described above in the two-stage setting; however, treatment selection is made at the end of the phase II component.

Table 10.1 summarises various requirements for the design of the trial, as well as the desirable practical elements associated with design selection (relating to software availability and early termination during phase II). Although none of the designs incorporate early termination for lack of activity *during* the phase II element, the design of Shun et al. does incorporate formal comparison with the control arm at the end of phase II, with a superiority comparison, as does the design of Todd and Stallard. Although the design of Todd and Stallard does not incorporate early schedule selection during phase II, the formal comparison between the control arm and each of

Table 10.1   Summary of practical considerations for each design.

Consideration	i	ii	iii	iv	v
Required					
Formal comparison with control	Y[a]	Y	Y	Y	Y
Two-stage phase II	Y	Y	N	N	N
Desirable					
Statistical software/programs available	N	N	Y	N	N
Early termination for lack of activity (*during* phase II)	N	N	N	N	N

[a]Non-superiority comparison.

the schedules to perform selection inherently makes the selection robust. Additionally, the design of Todd and Stallard clearly outlines the approach to the group-sequential phase III trial, incorporating multiple assessments of efficacy throughout the duration of the trial, and has software available. Due to the additional detail provided with this design and software availability, it was deemed appropriate to adopt the design of Todd and Stallard, building an additional interim assessment of safety and tolerability into the phase II element.

Proposed trial design

It is difficult to determine reliable estimates of PSA DT specifically for the cohort of men who, with their clinicians, would participate in a controlled trial of new treatment versus no immediate intervention (i.e. watchful waiting), since such a cohort is likely a very selected population of patients. On the assumption that men with doubling times of <8 months (or their clinicians) may be most likely to opt for treatment intervention and those with slow doubling times in excess of 12 months may decide they do not want any treatment at this stage, we estimate mean PSA DT with watchful waiting in the current trial to be approximately 8 months, with an associated standard deviation of 4 months. An increase in PSA DT of at least 4 months (50% increase), that is, average doubling time with vaccine C 12 months, is deemed worthy of further consideration in phase III. Under the design of Todd and Stallard, the standardised PSA DT difference between each schedule and the control arm will be used as the measure of treatment effect and corresponds to a target value of 1.0 (Todd and Stallard 2005). Using a 5% one-sided significance level and with 90% power, a total of 18 patients per arm are required in the phase II trial. Accounting for a 20% dropout rate, a total of 66 patients will be recruited (22 per arm) to the phase II component. Since the estimate of mean doubling time in the control arm is somewhat unreliable, an interim assessment during phase II will be conducted to evaluate whether an increase in sample size is required. This will be performed by an independent data monitoring committee. Additionally, ongoing assessments of safety and tolerability will be performed throughout the trial, with no formal stopping rules applied to these endpoints.

The trial is designed as a phase II/III trial using the group-sequential design of Todd and Stallard (2005). At the end of the phase II component, when patients have been followed up for at least 12 months to observe changes in PSA levels over time, a formal comparison between the two dosing schedules of vaccine C and the control arm of watchful waiting will be performed. A dosing schedule will be selected for further evaluation in the phase III component if there is a statistically significant increase in PSA DT of at least 50%. If neither of the dosing schedules pass this boundary, the trial may be terminated for lack of activity. Should both dosing schedules be found to significantly improve PSA DT, the schedule with the largest treatment effect estimate may be selected, and patients will continue to be randomised between the selected schedule and watchful waiting under the phase III component.

In this population of patients, median time to development of metastases is approximately 8 years (Pound et al. 1999). In the current trial, upon further biochemical progression after vaccine C or watchful waiting, patients may receive further treatment to include androgen-deprivation therapy. Due to the long follow-up times required to observe development of metastases, the phase III component is designed to detect a clinically relevant improvement in time from randomisation to androgen independence (TAI) with the use of the selected schedule of vaccine C, as the primary outcome measure. Time to development of metastases (TDM) will be incorporated as a long-term secondary endpoint. There is a paucity of data in this specific setting from which to determine TAI; however, it is anticipated that in this population of patients, the median time from androgen independence to distant metastases is approximately 30 months (Smith et al. 2005). A median time from randomisation to androgen independence for patients initially randomised to watchful waiting is therefore assumed to be approximately 66 months ($5\frac{1}{5}$ years). An improvement in median TAI of 1.4 years with vaccine C is deemed clinically relevant, corresponding to a hazard ratio of 0.8. A maximum of 1400 patients will be randomised to receive either watchful waiting or the selected schedule of vaccine C, with a single interim assessment for futility as described in detail by Todd and Stallard (2005), and accounting for dropout. This design also provides sufficient power to detect an improvement in median TDM from 8 to 10 years with vaccine C.

Summary

This trial has been designed to select an active dosing schedule of vaccine C to take forward into phase III evaluation, for patients with biochemical-failure-only prostate cancer. This phase II/III trial has been designed to reflect the practical issues associated with drug development in disease areas where long-term follow-up of patients is required to observe sufficient data for phase III registration studies. A statistically efficient phase II design has been identified to select the more active of two dosing regimens of vaccine C to take forward in to the phase III component.

Taking into account therapeutic considerations associated with the vaccine, the patient population, external literature regarding appropriate outcome measures in prostate cancer, available outcome measure data and the development pathway of

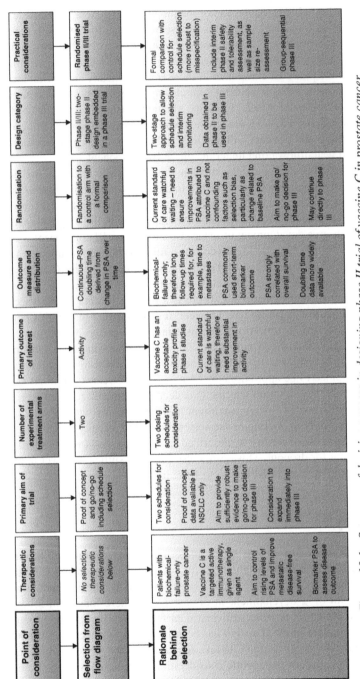

Figure 10.1 Summary of decision process in designing phase II trial of vaccine C in prostate cancer.

the vaccine, we addressed the trial-specific design requirements for each of the eight points featured in Figure 2.1 and described in Chapter 2, as summarised in Figure 10.1. Working through the thought process and taking an iterative approach to the design of the trial, with ongoing discussion between the clinician and statistician, we have designed a randomised, controlled, seamless phase II/III selection trial. Although the design does not meet the exact initial specifications (i.e. two-stage phase II), the iterative process and review of available designs further informed the decision process, resulting in an appropriate design, as determined by the trial team. This highlights the benefits of considering all available options and taking a practical approach to trial design. The design incorporates dose schedule selection via formal comparison with the current standard of care, watchful waiting, for the assessment of PSA DT, derived from changes in PSA levels over time, as the primary phase II outcome measure in biochemical-failure-only prostate cancer patients. Additionally, the phase III component incorporates group-sequential assessment of the phase III primary endpoint of time to androgen independence.

11

Dose selection in advanced multiple myeloma

Sarah Brown and Steve Schey

The outlook for patients with multiple myeloma relapsing after optimal therapy with thalidomide, lenalidomide and bortezomib is poor, and patients with disease refractory to initial treatments have an especially poor prognosis. There is no consensus on the optimal therapy for these patients. Drug D is a uniquely structured alkylating anti-tumour agent that lacks cross-resistance with other alkylating agents. There is very good evidence to show that combinations of an alkylator, thalidomide and corticosteroid are effective in treating patients with relapsed/refractory multiple myeloma (Facon et al. 2007; Palumbo et al. 2006, 2008). Drug D in combination with thalidomide and dexamethasone is therefore proposed as a combination therapy for phase II investigation in this population of patients. Data are available suggesting that drug D adds to the activity of other combination therapies; the optimal dose of drug D as combination therapy is not, however, known. A dose selection study is proposed to consider the optimal dose of drug D in combination with thalidomide and dexamethasone (DTD). A phase II selection study of DTD (dose 1) versus DTD (dose 2) is proposed.

Stage 1 – Trial questions

Therapeutic considerations

Mechanism of action: Drug D is an alkylating agent which, when given in combination with thalidomide and dexamethasone, is expected to induce disease response.

A Practical Guide to Designing Phase II Trials in Oncology, First Edition.
Sarah R. Brown, Walter M. Gregory, Chris Twelves and Julia Brown.
© 2014 John Wiley & Sons, Ltd. Published 2014 by John Wiley & Sons, Ltd.

Aim of treatment: The ultimate aim of treatment in this population of patients is to improve overall survival. Whilst it may be demonstrated that a drug may be active *ex vivo*, this is not of value unless it is at doses that can be achieved *in vivo*. Progression-free and event-free survival may also be desirable endpoints. Whilst activity can often be demonstrated *ex vivo*, for a drug to be effective as a treatment, it needs to be shown that the drug can be delivered in patients at the dose required without unacceptable toxicity. It is known from previous studies of similar treatments that patients may have difficulty receiving a full course of treatment due to cumulative haematological toxicities. Such cumulative toxicity, emerging in later cycles, may not be identified in phase I studies where the tolerability usually focuses on cycle 1. It is, therefore, important to demonstrate not only anti-tumour activity, indicating potential to improve overall survival, but also acceptable tolerability and the ability to deliver the treatment, when recommending an optimal dose.

Single or combination therapy: Drug D is to be given in combination with thalidomide and dexamethasone.

Biomarkers: Although aberrant expression of phenotypic, cytogenetic or molecular markers can be used to define poor prognosis disease, there are no agreed biomarkers consistently demonstrated to be associated with response or prognosis for drug D, or with regard to outcome measures of disease activity in this setting, to enable patient enrichment or alternative assessment of therapeutic activity. Paraprotein is used as a surrogate marker of tumour bulk in secretory myeloma whilst the serum-free light chains can be utilised in the less common light-chain myeloma or non-secretory disease. They are monitored serially during treatment to assess the response to treatment but are less sensitive than immunophenotyping in identifying minimal residual disease. Currently, there is a lack of robust, prospective data for the use of alternative biomarkers but validation studies are ongoing.

Primary intention of trial

The primary objective of the study is to identify a dose of drug D given in combination with dexamethasone and thalidomide that is active and tolerable and can be consistently delivered to patients with relapsed/refractory multiple myeloma, with the intention of taking that combination forward into studies in newly diagnosed patients. A randomised phase II selection trial incorporating proof of concept for the de novo study is therefore proposed.

Number of experimental arms

Although there is only one experimental drug under investigation, there are two doses of drug D being considered. There are, therefore, two experimental arms.

Primary outcome of interest

Drug D, and other similar drugs used to treat myeloma, may be associated with cumulative toxicity. It is important to demonstrate that drug D in combination with thalidomide and dexamethasone is both sufficiently active and tolerable, in terms of being deliverable; therefore, an assessment of tolerability is incorporated as a primary outcome measure in this trial. This is seen as being equally as important as demonstrating activity, therefore joint primary outcome measures of toxicity/tolerability and activity will be used.

Stage 2 – Design components

Outcome measure and distribution

The tolerability of DTD may be measured by the ability to deliver drug D in full dose and on time for at least two cycles, that is, a binary outcome measure. If a patient is unable to receive the first two cycles of treatment without any haematological toxicities requiring dose delay or reduction, this is an indication that there are likely to be future tolerability issues with the combination, requiring dose reductions or delays.

Drug D is a cytotoxic agent expected to induce disease response. There are, unfortunately, limited data regarding the use of surrogate endpoints associated with overall survival in relapsed refractory multiple myeloma patients. However, overall response rate, in combination with substantial response duration, has been recommended as an appropriate endpoint for accelerated approval of new myeloma agents by the US Food and Drug Administration (Anderson et al. 2005), and response rates (complete response plus partial response) have been recommended as benchmark outcomes in trials in the relapsed and refractory setting (Anderson et al. 2007). It was therefore deemed appropriate to base the assessment of activity on the outcome measure of partial response or, better, a binary outcome measure assessed over up to six cycles of treatment with DTD.

Dual primary outcome measures of activity and tolerability will be assessed using the endpoints of partial response or better and ability to tolerate at least two cycles of treatment, respectively.

Randomisation

Randomisation will be performed between DTD (dose 1) and DTD (dose 2), for the purpose of dose selection. Although drug D is to be given in combination with both thalidomide and dexamethasone, there is no standard therapy available for this population of patients.

As previously highlighted, the aim of the current trial is to identify a dose of drug D in combination with thalidomide and dexamethasone that is sufficiently active and tolerable to warrant investigation in the de novo setting. It is expected that the subsequent study in the de novo setting would be a further randomised trial, with a conventional control arm to establish the benefit, or otherwise, from drug D administered at an optimal dose in combination with thalidomide and dexamethasone compared to 'standard therapy'. As such, no conventional 'control' arm is incorporated in the current trial, since the aim of the study is not to quantify the benefit, or otherwise, of drug D in combination with thalidomide and dexamethasone, over and above a current standard therapy, but to provide proof of concept data.

Historical control data are available from two large randomised phase III studies in a similar population of patients, providing initial data on which to base the assumptions made within the current trial.

Design category

Rejected designs:

i. Upon discussion with the clinical investigators, it was decided that assessing the data early in the trial was important to ensure the tolerability of the treatment is not too low and that the activity is sufficiently high. A one-stage design was therefore rejected.

ii. Due to the nature of the primary activity outcome measure assessed over up to six cycles of treatment, final response results will not be available until 6 months after randomisation. For logistical reasons a multi-stage or continuous monitoring design was deemed inappropriate, as they require data to be available in a 'real-time' manner.

iii. As already noted, the follow-on study is expected to be in a different setting to the current study, that is, de novo versus heavily pre-treated; therefore a seamless phase II/III study would not be possible.

iv. Decision-theoretic approaches to trial design require information on number of patients to be treated in future phase III trials, total patient horizon (number of patients in the population who may potentially be treated with the new drug were it approved) and costs of treatment. Since the subsequent study is expected to be in a different setting, with different decision-theoretic parameters, such an approach is again not appropriate.

v. A three-outcome design, which allows an 'inconclusive' result to be identified for the primary endpoint, and additional, secondary, endpoints to be taken into account, was also deemed inappropriate since a dual primary endpoint is already being considered.

vi. Finally, randomised discontinuation designs were also considered but rejected since the study does not aim to determine the additional benefit of drug D over thalidomide and dexamethasone. Moreover, a discontinuation design does not suit a study aimed at evaluating different doses of a study drug.

Candidate designs: Two-stage designs were considered as potential designs for the trial.

Possible designs

On the basis of the above exclusions and the requirement to assess tolerability and activity at an interim time point, a two-stage trial design was chosen, incorporating dose selection between DTD (dose 1) and DTD (dose 2), to select an optimal dose of drug D in a subsequent study of DTD in the de novo setting. The trial will incorporate joint primary outcome measures of toxicity/tolerability and activity.

It is possible to conduct selection trials designed with go/no-go decision criteria that are applied to each individual arm, to ensure that only those arms sufficiently active (and tolerable), that is, passing the 'go' criteria, are compared for selection, as opposed to simply selecting the dose with the better activity and tolerability. Such an approach is described by Simon et al. (1985) and Sargent and Goldberg (2001), in the context of binary outcomes, and will be considered here.

There are no two-stage designs for dual-endpoint selection trials described in Section 6.4, which fit the design parameters described above; however, the following multi-stage design may be considered:

i. Thall and Sung (1998) – multi-stage design which may be adapted to incorporate just two stages

Additionally, applying the concept of Simon et al. (1985) or Sargent and Goldberg (2001), the following two-stage designs for dual-endpoint single-arm trials may also be considered (Section 6.2):

ii. Bryant and Day (1995)

iii. Conaway and Petroni (1995)

iv. Conaway and Petroni (1996)

v. Thall and Cheng (2001)

vi. Jin (2007)

vii. Wu and Liu (2007)

Stage 3 – Practicalities

Practical considerations for selecting between designs

We now consider each of the above designs in turn.

Dual-endpoint selection designs

i. Thall and Sung propose a Bayesian multi-stage design, which may be reduced to incorporate just two stages, to assess multiple outcomes, for example, toxicity and activity. They specifically outline application of this design to randomised phase II selection trials. Outcomes are categorised into k levels (e.g. active/not toxic; active/toxic; not active/toxic; not active/not toxic) and priors based on historical data. Clinicians need to provide information on the trade-off between activity and toxicity, that is, the acceptable increase in toxicity for a specific increase in activity. The joint probability of both a response and toxicity, often specified in terms of a conditional probability or an odds ratio, should be accounted for when assessing the operating characteristics of the design.

The impact of this relationship between activity and toxicity was investigated via example, varying the odds ratio between the probability of toxicity when response occurs, relative to no response. The operating characteristics were not sensitive to the relationship specified. Selection may be based on any appropriate criterion applied at the end of the trial to those treatments not terminated early due to unacceptably high toxicity or unacceptably low activity (in the case where there is more than one treatment passing the first stage). As an example, selection may be based on the treatment with the highest response rate and toxicity below a specific level, from those treatments not terminated early. Software is available to allow implementation of the design.

Dual-endpoint single-arm designs (i.e. incorporating selection after assessment of each individual arm)

ii. Bryant and Day propose a design that reflects that of Simon's two-stage design for a single outcome measure (Simon 1989). Early termination for unacceptably low activity or unacceptably high toxicity is incorporated at the end of the first stage. The design assumes toxicity and activity are independent. This is arguably unlikely to be the case for most trials; however, the impact of incorrectly assuming independence was assessed and the design found to be reasonably insensitive to this. Software is available to enable implementation.

iii. Conaway and Petroni (1995) propose a design based on enumerating the exact distribution for two binary endpoints. Estimation of the association between the activity and toxicity outcomes is required, for example, in the form of the correlation or an odds ratio. Early termination for unacceptably low activity or unacceptably high toxicity is incorporated at the end of the first stage. The authors note that the design, with respect to power, is robust against misspecification of the association parameter. Programs to enable implementation are noted as being available from the author.

iv. The design proposed by Conaway and Petroni in 1996 incorporates assessment of toxicity and activity based on the I-divergence test statistic incorporating all four combinations of toxicity and activity described previously, allowing a trade-off between activity and toxicity. This differs from their previous design (Conaway and Petroni 1995) and the Bryant and Day design, which base results on the overall activity and toxicity rates. An estimate of the association between activity and toxicity is required; however, the authors note that the properties of the test are reasonably unaffected by misspecification. Early termination for unacceptably low activity or unacceptably high toxicity is incorporated at the end of the first stage. Programs are not noted as being available from the authors; therefore, the design may need programming for implementation.

v. The design proposed by Thall and Cheng, in the setting with no control arm, allows for assessment of improvement in activity with the experimental treatment whilst *not increasing* toxicity, compared to historical control data. No discussion is provided regarding the correlation between the endpoints and robustness to misspecification of this relationship. The design would require programming to enable implementation.

vi. Jin proposed an alternative test to that of Conaway and Petroni (1996), designed to deal with trade-off between toxicity and activity by controlling the marginal type I errors for these two outcomes separately. Incorporating this additional control inevitably increases sample size. As for other designs, an estimate of the association between the two outcome measures is required, and the design is robust to misspecification with regard to statistical power. Early termination for unacceptably low activity or unacceptably high toxicity is incorporated at the end of the first stage. This design would need programming to enable implementation.

vii. Wu and Liu propose an adaptation to the designs proposed by, for example, Conaway and Petroni (1995). The adaptation incorporates a sample size readjustment at the end of the first stage to allow for inaccuracy in the initial specification of the association between activity and toxicity. In this respect, the interim assessment focuses on sample size re-estimation rather than early termination for lack of activity or unacceptable toxicity. Programming requirements are as for the original designs.

In the case of designs (ii)–(vii), the focus is to determine activity and tolerability of each of the experimental regimens individually. In the case where both regimens are found to be sufficiently tolerable and active, additional secondary selection criteria should be employed.

Table 11.1 provides a summary of the practical considerations for each design. There are a number of designs in this example that are appropriate to the specific requirements of the trial. Taking a practical approach for the purpose of this example, we consider only those which are deemed robust to misspecification of the relationship between the endpoints and for which software is available. This includes the following designs: (i) Thall and Sung, (ii) Bryant and Day and (iii) Conaway and Petroni. In reality, further exploration of the designs for which no software is available is also recommended.

Table 11.1   Summary of practical considerations for each design.

Consideration	i	ii	iii	iv	v	vi	vii
Required							
Robust to misspecification of relationship between endpoints	Y	Y	Y	Y	Not discussed	Y	Y
Desirable							
Statistical software/ programs available	Y	Y	Y	N	N	N	N/A[a]

[a]Availability according to the original methods from which the sample size is adopted.

Tournoux et al. (2007) compared the designs of Bryant and Day (1995) and Conaway and Petroni (1995). The Bryant and Day design was more robust to misspecification of the relationship between activity and toxicity. We may therefore choose between the Bayesian design of Thall and Sung which incorporates treatment selection and the frequentist design of Bryant and Day which requires the use of additional, secondary, selection procedures. Again taking a practical approach for the purpose of this example, we present here the proposed trial design based on the design described by Bryant and Day; however, the design presented by Thall and Sung may equally be considered.

Using the Bryant and Day design requires the inclusion of an additional, secondary, selection approach should both dosing schedules be found to be sufficiently active and tolerable. Such designs are described by Simon et al. (1985) and Sargent and Goldberg (2001) and are discussed in Chapter 5. In the current setting we propose to perform selection on the basis of PFS, using the design of Sargent and Goldberg. This design selects the dosing schedule with the higher PFS rate with a derived probability of correct selection *only* when the difference in PFS between the two schedules is larger than a pre-specified value. In the case where the difference is less than this, selection may be based on alternative criteria. This differs to the design described by Simon et al. which will always select a schedule with higher PFS, regardless of the magnitude of difference between the two arms, thus potentially leading to increased probability of incorrect selection.

Proposed trial design

We first consider the design for each dosing schedule individually, before moving to regimen selection. Previously published data in a slightly less pre-treated population of patients are available to provide estimates of historical control data (van de Donk et al. 2011). Overall response rates were 60%. Since the population of patients in the current trial is expected to be more heavily pre-treated than those in the previous studies, a response rate of at least 50% with drug D in combination with TD is targeted. A response rate of 20% is taken as the response rate below which a dosing combination would be rejected. Considering tolerability rates, previous data identified 20% of patients unable to tolerate treatment. For the purpose of the current trial, a tolerability rate of 75% or less, that is, >25% intolerable, is taken to be unacceptable and would lead to a recommendation of rejecting the dosing combination. A tolerability rate of 90% is targeted with this regimen, that is, 10% intolerability, a relative reduction of 50% compared to historical control data, deemed clinically relevant.

After discussion with the clinicians it was agreed that the trial should be designed with 90% power and 10% type I error rates for both activity and tolerability (i.e. 10% chance that a dosing schedule is deemed active when in fact the response rate is <20% and 10% chance a dosing schedule is deemed tolerable when in fact tolerability is <75%). Implementing this design using software provided by Machin et al. (2008), the corresponding design is as follows, for each arm separately.

- Stage 1: Recruit 20 patients and follow up to observe response and tolerability. If at least 4/20 patients achieve a response *and* at least 15/20 patients are able to tolerate treatment, continue to stage 2. If there are three or fewer patients who do not achieve a response, the dosing schedule is terminated early for lack of activity; if there are 14 or fewer patients who are able to tolerate treatment, the dosing schedule is terminated early for non-tolerability.

- Stage 2: Recruit a further 24 patients to a total of 44 in each arm. Follow up to observe response and tolerability. If at least 13/44 patients achieve a response *and* at least 36/44 patients are able to tolerate treatment, the dosing schedule is deemed sufficiently active and tolerable. If there are 12 or fewer patients who do not achieve a response, the dosing schedule is rejected for lack of activity; if there are 35 or fewer patients who are able to tolerate treatment, the dosing schedule is rejected for non-tolerability.

If only one of the dosing schedules successfully passes stage 2, this dosing schedule will be selected for further investigation. In the case where both dosing schedules successfully pass stage 2 and are deemed sufficiently active and tolerable to warrant further investigation, the selection criteria of Sargent and Goldberg are applied, as previously described. It was agreed that the dosing schedule with the higher PFS rate at 12 months should be selected only when the difference in 12-month PFS rates between the two arms is greater than 5%. A 25% PFS rate at 12 months with dose 1 and a 35% PFS rate with dose 2 were hypothesised based on previously published data for drug D. With 44 patients per arm and observed PFS rates of 25% and 35% in the dose 1 and 2 arms, respectively, the study would correctly select the dose schedule with higher PFS rate with 81% probability (assuming that in 50% of ambiguous cases the correct treatment would be selected), based on PFS alone. If the difference is less than 5%, alternative selection criteria may be considered.

Patients will be randomised on a 1:1 basis to receive either DTD (dose 1) or DTD (dose 2), with a maximum of 88 patients randomised (44 per arm).

Summary

This trial has been designed to select the best dosing schedule of a cytotoxic agent, drug D, when given in combination with thalidomide and dexamethasone in patients with relapsed refractory multiple myeloma. Sufficient activity and tolerability of dose 1 and dose 2 are initially incorporated to select between the two doses, with additional, secondary, selection only in the case where both dosing schedules are found sufficiently active and tolerable. Schedule selection is then determined on the basis of progression-free survival.

By taking into account therapeutic considerations associated with the drug, the patient population and available historical control data and taking pragmatic approaches to trial design, the specific design criteria associated with each of the

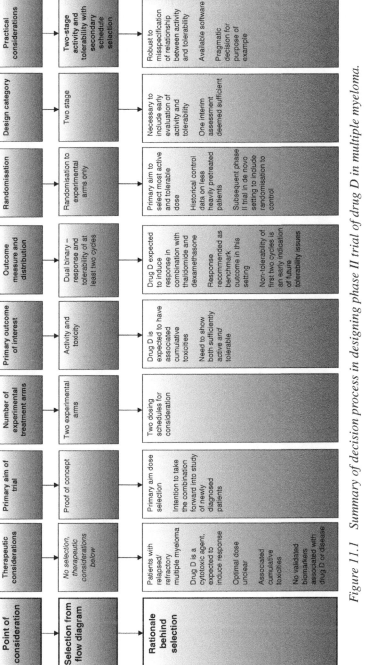

Figure 11.1   Summary of decision process in designing phase II trial of drug D in multiple myeloma.

eight elements featured in Figure 2.1 and described in Chapter 2 are summarised in Figure 11.1. Working through the thought process and taking an iterative approach to the design of the trial, with ongoing discussion between the clinician and statistician, we have designed a randomised, phase II selection trial, for the selection of the optimal dose of drug D in combination with thalidomide and dexamethasone (DTD) in patients with relapsed refractory multiple myeloma.

12

Targeted therapy for advanced colorectal cancer

Matthew Seymour and Sarah Brown

Drug E is a monoclonal antibody therapy targeting a cell surface receptor, 'Receptor X', that is known to be involved in cell growth from some cancers. Retrospective studies have shown that Receptor X is strongly expressed in around 5% of colorectal cancers, and it is now hypothesised that drug E, given in combination with current standard chemotherapy, will improve efficacy for patients with X-positive advanced colorectal cancer (aCRC) after failure of first-line chemotherapy. Receptor X is not routinely measured in aCRC, so there are only limited historical data from previous trials on which to base the expected control outcomes in this specific group. Phase III clinical data are available for the efficacy of drug E in other solid tumours where Receptor X is more commonly expressed, and it is hoped that a similar treatment effect will occur in X-positive aCRC. Drug E has demonstrated an acceptable toxicity profile in studies in other disease areas. A phase II trial of drug E in combination with standard second-line chemotherapy, for Receptor-X-positive aCRC patients, is proposed to determine whether to proceed to a larger phase III trial.

Stage 1 – Trial questions

Therapeutic considerations

Mechanism of action: Drug E is a monoclonal antibody directed against Receptor X. It is believed to be primarily cytostatic as a single agent, but to act synergistically

A Practical Guide to Designing Phase II Trials in Oncology, First Edition.
Sarah R. Brown, Walter M. Gregory, Chris Twelves and Julia Brown.
© 2014 John Wiley & Sons, Ltd. Published 2014 by John Wiley & Sons, Ltd.

with standard cytotoxic chemotherapy. In the setting of second-line treatment for aCRC, classical cytotoxic chemotherapies are associated with low response rates due to high levels of tumour resistance. It is, therefore, unrealistic to expect the addition of drug E to chemotherapy to induce a high response rate. An assessment of disease control, that is, progression-free survival (PFS), offers a more realistic measure of the efficacy of this combination in this setting.

Aim of treatment: The ultimate aim of second-line treatment of patients with advanced disease is to prolong overall survival. An early indicator of treatment activity is the ability to prolong PFS, as discussed above.

Single or combination therapy: Drug E is given in combination with standard second-line chemotherapy; to be relevant, therefore, the activity of the combination therapy would need to be greater than that of chemotherapy alone.

Biomarkers: Drug E targets the specific cell surface receptor, Receptor X, so the trial will be focused specifically on patients with X-positive tumours. On the basis of evidence in other disease areas, the drug is not expected to improve clinical outcomes in patients with X-negative tumours; these patients will, therefore, be excluded. There are no validated biomarkers associated with aCRC which may provide an alternative assessment of therapeutic activity.

Primary intention of trial

There is confirmed clinical evidence of efficacy of drug E in other solid tumours (breast and gastrointestinal cancer). Owing to the small population of patients available, the current phase II trial is designed to deliver proof of concept in this targeted population of patients and a go/no-go decision for a subsequent phase III trial. It is important to consider the most efficient trial designs due to the rarity of the target population, as well as the length of time required for a drug to move from phase II to phase III then into routine clinical practice. A pragmatic approach to designing trials in these settings is essential, to ensure reliable and robust trial design, whilst maintaining an efficient and achievable drug development pathway.

Number of experimental treatment arms

There is only one experimental treatment under investigation, so a selection trial is not required.

Primary outcome of interest

Drug E has shown an acceptable toxicity profile in multiple studies in other solid tumours. The current combination in aCRC is expected to have only minimal additional toxicity or functional deficit. While toxicity will form a secondary endpoint of the phase II trial, the primary outcome of interest is activity.

Stage 2 – Design components

Outcome measure and distribution

In this heavily pre-treated population of patients, response rates to chemotherapy are historically low and the addition of drug E is not expected to induce a high response rate. The use of PFS as an indicator of activity may, therefore, be more appropriate and clinically relevant. PFS is strongly correlated with overall survival in patients with aCRC (Buyse et al. 2007), albeit predominantly in the setting of trials of chemotherapeutic agents.

Chemotherapy plus drug E will be given for an initial period of 12 weeks, reflecting the initial treatment period of standard chemotherapy. After this point, patients who have not progressed will continue to receive drug E until progression. Assessments of disease status via CT scan will be carried out approximately 12-weekly until disease progression. Median PFS with standard chemotherapy is approximately 4.8 months in patients with advanced colorectal cancer following first-line therapy, but data specifically for patients with X-positive colorectal cancer are limited (see Section 12.4 for further details). This population of patients represents a rare subgroup of aCRC patients, so recruitment to the study will likely be slow. A binary outcome dichotomising PFS at a single time point (i.e. the proportion of patients free of disease progression at a specific time point) is worthy of consideration due to the long period of recruitment and the requirement otherwise for all patients to be followed up to disease progression. If inclusion of interim assessments during the trial is being considered, however, the requirement to wait for all patients to be followed up to the specific time point of interest before this can take place may be impractical. The use of all time-to-event data up to and including the specific time point may be considered a possibility in this setting. Conversely, PFS will be limited and the use of a time-to-event outcome (i.e. overall PFS) may be preferable since this incorporates all available information from the trial and will further facilitate design of the potential phase III trial that would have a time-to-event primary outcome measure.

Randomisation

Drug E is to be given in combination with standard chemotherapy. It is important that any possible additional activity observed with the combination can reasonably be attributed to the addition of drug E. In the absence of reliable historical control data for this population of patients with X-positive aCRC, randomisation should be incorporated to provide robust and reliable results. Randomisation will increase the number of patients required with what is a rare sub-type of a more common cancer, so it is also important to minimise the sample size in other ways. Since the trial is being designed to provide sufficient data to determine whether to progress to a phase III trial, randomisation is essential despite its impact on patient numbers. A key consideration is the incorporation, or otherwise, of formal statistical comparison with control. While this is preferable for the purpose of making a stop/go decision, to sufficiently power such a comparison with an acceptable type I error rate may be prohibitive within such a rare population. On the other hand, an additional consideration is the targeted treatment effect with the experimental treatment. In studies adding drug E to standard chemotherapy in other disease areas, hazard ratios of between 0.5 and 0.7 have been observed. When such large treatment effects are realistic, it may be feasible to perform formal statistical comparisons between experimental and control arms, with limited sample sizes.

Randomisation will, therefore, be incorporated, and the feasibility of including a formally powered comparison with a control will be considered, with regard to impact on sample size. Should drug E show a sufficient level of activity, a subsequent randomised phase III trial with multiple interim assessments for lack of efficacy is envisaged.

Design category

Especially where historical data may be unreliable it is important to consider multiple scenarios when choosing the statistical design, to assess how robust each design is if outcomes in either treatment arm are not as expected. For example, if activity in the control arm is uncertain, how well do the different trial designs cope with an under- or over-estimation of this activity?

Rejected designs:

i. Decision-theoretic approaches to trial design incorporate information on number of patients to be treated in future phase III trials, number of patients potentially benefitting from future treatment and costs of treatment. In this particular setting, the costs associated with the current treatment are expected to change in the near future due to patent expiry. The data are, therefore, not reliable for the purpose of a decision-theoretic design and this design was deemed inappropriate.

ii. Randomised discontinuation designs were also rejected, on the basis that the initial assessment of treatment activity is carried out on completion of the first block of combination treatment, after which treatment is with single agent drug E only. Although it may be possible for all patients to receive initial treatment with drug E plus chemotherapy, to randomise patients free of progression at 12 weeks to drug E versus no treatment is not the central question here. Rather, the trial is designed to address the treatment schedule as a whole, that is, initial combination therapy followed by single-agent maintenance therapy, compared with chemotherapy alone, so a randomisation discontinuation design was rejected.

iii. Due to the rarity of the subgroup of patients considered in this trial, and the potential subsequent phase III trial, seamless phase II/III designs were deemed inappropriate given the uncertainty regarding feasibility of recruiting large numbers of patients.

iv. Studies in other solid tumours have shown large treatment effects, with hazard ratios in the region of 0.5–0.7 with the addition of drug E to standard chemotherapy. With the addition of this monoclonal antibody to current standard chemotherapy, there is no reason to expect that toxicity will be reduced (although neither is it expected that significant additional toxicities will emerge), and the combination therapy will ultimately be more costly than standard chemotherapy alone. A three-outcome design which enables alternative outcome measures such as toxicity and cost to be considered in the event that the treatment effect is inconclusive (i.e. it lies within a 'grey area' between declaring the treatment worthy of further investigation and not worthy of further investigation) is not appropriate here since we do not expect either of these measures to be reduced with the use of drug E.

v. As previously noted, the proportion of aCRC patients with X-positive disease is low; therefore, recruitment is expected to be relatively slow. The ability to build in early stopping boundaries for lack of activity is beneficial in this setting due to the potentially prolonged period of recruitment. On this basis two-stage designs were felt preferable to one-stage designs that do not incorporate formal interim assessment and the opportunity for early cessation. The use of a multi-stage design, or a continuous monitoring design, was considered but a single interim assessment was considered sufficient provided recruitment could continue during the stage 1 analysis as the eligible patient population is small and it is important not to 'lose' potential patients due to a halt in recruitment.

Candidate designs: Two-stage designs were considered as potential designs for the trial.

Possible designs

We have determined that the phase II trial will be a randomised trial, addressing both the proof of concept of drug E in combination with standard chemotherapy and the decision to proceed or not to phase III, on the basis of activity alone. This will be assessed using the time-to-event outcome measure of PFS, either incorporating all available data on PFS or enabling all available data up to and including a specific time point to be incorporated. Thus we consider designs listed under time-to-event outcome measures only. A two-stage statistical design will be used. Inclusion of randomisation for the purpose of formally powered statistical comparison will be addressed by taking a pragmatic approach to the necessary sample size in the context of the target population being small but the potential treatment effect large. Single-arm designs which enable randomisation for the purpose of calibration only, as well as randomised designs incorporating formally powered comparison, are therefore considered. Designs are identified from Chapter 3, single-arm trial designs that are adapted to include a randomised reference arm, or from Chapter 4.

Reviewing the available designs in Chapters 3 and 4 which fit these design parameters, the following designs may be considered for this trial. Discussion as to selecting between these specific designs is given in the next section.

From Chapter 3

 i. Case and Morgan (2003)

 ii. Litwin et al. (2007)

Although there are no two-stage designs listed in Chapter 4 with time-to-event endpoints, the principles of, for example, Herson and Carter (1986) or Buyse (2000) may be incorporated into the designs listed above, to assess the credibility of the outcome in the experimental arm. Alternatively, the one-stage designs from Chapter 4 noted below may be considered, with an adaptation to incorporate an interim assessment for lack of activity:

 iii. Stone et al. (2007b) and Simon et al. (2001)

 iv. Chen and Beckman (2009)

Stage 3 – Practicalities

Practical considerations for selecting between designs

We now consider each of the above designs in turn.

 i. The design proposed by Case and Morgan incorporates a time-to-event outcome measure whereby all information available at the time of the interim analysis is included. This is achieved by identifying a specific time point of interest at which the probability of PFS is assessed, in other words, a binary outcome derived from the time-to-event outcome incorporating all available data, including those patients with follow-up to less than the time point of interest. This design does not require a halt to recruitment. Standard programs are available for this design. Although a control arm may be included for the purpose of calibration, this does not power the study for formal comparison of the arms.

 ii. The design of Litwin et al. is based on a time-to-event outcome measure at two specific time points, that is, a binary outcome. This design does not incorporate data for patients who have not yet been followed up to the specific time point of interest at the interim assessment, and is therefore not considered further.

 iii. Stone and colleagues describe a phase II design which is formally powered to compare the experimental arm with the control arm, using relaxed type I errors and potentially targeting large treatment effects. This reflects the designs described by Simon in the setting of time-to-event outcomes, which are described by the authors as 'phase 2.5 screening' designs, due to the use of phase III-type designs but with type I error rates typically associated with phase II trials (Simon et al. 2001). By incorporating a formally powered statistical comparison with the control arm, the sample size of the trial will inevitably increase. This should, however, be weighed against the reliability of the decision-making criteria and compared with that for the non-comparative phase II design described in (i) above. Standard software is available for this design.

iv. Chen and Beckman describe an approach to a randomised phase II trial design that incorporates the ratio of sample sizes between phases II and III. Optimal type I and II errors for the design are identified by means of an efficiency score function. Formal comparison with the control arm is incorporated. The design considers cost efficiency of the phase II and III trials based on the ratio of sample sizes between phases II and III and the *a priori* probability of success of the investigational treatment, to determine the sample size for phase II. Sufficient detail is provided within the paper to allow implementation and an R program is provided to identify optimal designs. At this stage, however, the design of the potential phase III trial is unclear, since the phase II study is designed in part to provide data on feasibility of recruitment with such a rare subgroup of patients. The design of Chen and Beckman is, therefore, not considered further.

To distinguish between the designs incorporating no formal comparison (Case and Morgan 2003) versus formal comparison (Stone et al. 2007b), we consider below the required sample sizes, bearing in mind the need to include an interim assessment for lack of activity using the design of Stone et al.

Proposed trial design

The primary assessment of activity is based on PFS. The trial is designed for patients with X-positive aCRC after failure of first-line chemotherapy. It is anticipated that approximately 30% of patients will have progressed on first-line therapy; for these patients the estimated median PFS with standard second-line chemotherapy is 2.6 months (Sobrero et al. 2008). The remaining 70% of patients are expected to have progressed during a treatment break, or on intermittent therapy, with first-line chemotherapy; the estimated median PFS for these patients treated with standard 're-challenge' chemotherapy is 5.7 months (Adams et al. 2011). It is acknowledged that the standard chemotherapy may, therefore, differ between these two groups of patients. The expected median PFS of patients after first-line therapy in the current trial is approximately 4.8 months since we have no evidence that Receptor X status is prognostic of outcome. In other disease areas, a reduction in hazard rate for PFS of 30–50% has been observed with the addition of drug E to chemotherapy. In the current setting, a hazard ratio of 0.6 is targeted (i.e. a reduction in hazard rate of 40%) with the addition of drug E to standard chemotherapy. This corresponds to a targeted median PFS of 8 months in the experimental arm.

The design of Case and Morgan requires a specific time point at which to assess the progression-free probability; we select the 24-week time point. Corresponding expected PFS probabilities at 24 weeks (5.5 months) post-randomisation are 45.2% in the control arm (i.e. a probability of progression that would not be of further interest) and 62.1% in the experimental arm (i.e. a probability of progression worthy of further investigation).

We assume that patients are to be recruited over no more than a 3-year period as more protracted recruitment risks loss of engagement from investigators and the potential that the clinical question behind the trial will have changed if other new treatments have become available. Power of 80% is selected to detect the targeted treatment effect, with a 10% one-sided type I error for incorrectly declaring the addition of drug E to standard chemotherapy worthy of further investigation.

Under the design of Case and Morgan we would require 51 patients in the experimental arm, with an interim analysis taking place after 23 patients are recruited, not accounting for dropout. This is based on minimising the expected duration of accrual under the null hypothesis (Case and Morgan 2003). In order to incorporate randomisation to a reference arm a 1:1 randomisation would simply double the sample size. Alternatively, an imbalanced randomisation such as 2:1 in favour of the experimental arm may be favoured in this setting where the specific population of patients is rare. This will provide sufficient data in the experimental arm whilst also guarding against selection bias. It retains a reference arm against which the control arm assumptions may be informally compared, but the design is not powered for formal statistical comparison between the arms. In this particular example, including a 2:1 randomisation between standard chemotherapy plus drug E and standard chemotherapy alone without formal statistical comparison, a total of up to 77 patients will be recruited (assuming successfully passing stage 1; chemotherapy plus drug E $n = 51$, chemotherapy alone $n = 26$).

Under the design of Stone et al., we would require 40 patients per arm, that is, a total of 80 patients, assuming all patients are followed up until disease progression and for a minimum of 6 months. An interim assessment for lack of activity, based on the design of Gehan (1961), would be incorporated to enable early termination of the trial in the event that the PFS probability at 24 weeks post-randomisation is not sufficiently large enough in the experimental arm, to warrant continuation.

Comparing the two designs, we can see that the inclusion of formal comparison between the arms increases the required sample size only marginally in this setting. This is because the design of Stone et al. considers all the time-to-event data through the 3 years of recruitment and additional follow-up, whereas the design of Case and Morgan, although taking into account the time-to-event data prior to the 24-week time point, focuses on the survival probabilities at 24 weeks. The inclusion of the additional data under the design of Stone et al. makes this a feasible approach in this particular setting with a long recruitment period and a large targeted treatment effect. Additionally, the inclusion of a formally powered statistical comparison between treatment arms is more robust to uncertainty in the estimation of activity of the control arm, at the design stage. This trial would therefore require approximately 1600 patients to be screened over 3 years to identify 80 patients with X-positive aCRC.

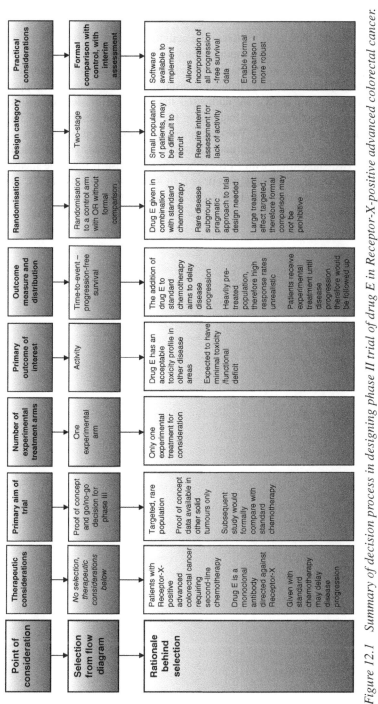

Figure 12.1 Summary of decision process in designing phase II trial of drug E in Receptor-X-positive advanced colorectal cancer.

Summary

This trial has been designed to assess the activity of the addition of a monoclonal antibody, drug E, to standard chemotherapy in patients with Receptor-X-positive aCRC. By taking into account therapeutic considerations associated with the drug, the rare patient population and mechanistic considerations associated with appropriate outcome measures in aCRC, we addressed the trial-specific design requirements through each of the three stages featured in Figure 2.1 and described in Chapter 2, as summarised in Figure 12.1. Working through the thought process with ongoing discussion between the clinician and statistician, we have designed a randomised, controlled, two-stage trial, with PFS as the primary phase II outcome measure for the assessment of chemotherapy plus drug E in Receptor-X-positive aCRC patients. The trial is designed to provide both proof of concept data and a go/no-go decision regarding whether or not to proceed to a larger randomised phase III trial.

13

Phase II oncology trials: Perspective from industry

Anthony Rossini, Steven Green and William Mietlowski

13.1 Introduction

In oncology clinical development, phase II has the widest range of possible goals which can be addressed at this stage. In contrast, there is general agreement for what is to be done at phase I and phase III. Phase I generates the initial data used to select a dose which can be used relatively safely in a larger population. Likewise, phase III studies aim to establish evidence justifying efficacy and safety enabling health authority approval. Generally, these designs focus on clinically relevant survival and event-time endpoints. Phase II trials, on the other hand, have the simple but ill-defined mission of providing evidence for one or more of the many possible strategic paths between these two phases. Specifically, the phase II programme must bridge between the current knowledge about the initially established dosing regimen and the phase III design to support registration. There are many possible paths, representing the many approaches to learning about how to use a compound to treat cancer. The diversity of clinical development paths can also be deduced from the range of clinical trial designs described in this book. This chapter will focus on selecting phase II designs originating in response to strategies embodied in a commercially oriented clinical development plan (CDP).

Commercially sponsored trials are a component of a pre-specified, evolving, comprehensive CDP. A CDP can be formally thought of as a document which frames the development of a compound in terms of medical indications, staging of activities

A Practical Guide to Designing Phase II Trials in Oncology, First Edition.
Sarah R. Brown, Walter M. Gregory, Chris Twelves and Julia Brown.
© 2014 John Wiley & Sons, Ltd. Published 2014 by John Wiley & Sons, Ltd.

and collection of data for justifying registration across possible indications. This contains justification for components which the development team considers essential to develop the compound. The choice of trial designs should address the CDP's objectives, conditional on previous results. The goal of the CDP is to provide a roadmap of activities to efficiently either deliver a commercially viable product or terminate development early for futility and/or safety issues. A commercially viable product requires both regulatory approval and agreement by payers to reimburse.

The selection process described in this chapter takes into account pharmaceutical drug development challenges and drivers. These frame the constraints and requirements which inform the selection of the phase II design(s). The source for these challenges arise both internally and externally and relate to both scientific and operational considerations. Internal clinical development decisions which impact phase II include timing and prioritisation of the compound in relation to other compounds in the portfolio. External clinical constraints and drivers include current medical practice, payer approaches and competition from external compounds. Constraints include both financial resources and shared internal specialised employee skills which are in limited supply and required for more sophisticated designs. Some parts of this chapter are forward looking and represent practices which are not yet incorporated. Other parts are retrospective and may be suboptimal or obsolete due to recent statistical, clinical or regulatory landscape changes. This chapter just reflects a snapshot in time of current thinking.

Multiple options often exist for clinical development strategies at the planning stage for the phase II programme, with acceleration and hesitation pressure coming from both the development team and the external environment. The selection of one or more strategies in the face of uncertainty informs the choice of phase II design(s) to be implemented. The range of strategic goals that are addressed in this chapter consists of those for potential registration, establishing exploratory activity, regimen selection, prediction of phase III success, safety trials and prospective identification of targeted populations. We next describe some of the commercial challenges and drivers before discussing strategic considerations and how they can inform study design selection.

13.2 Commercial challenges, drivers and considerations

The environment for commercial clinical drug development can change frequently, making fixed as well as long-term planning difficult. New information arises regarding science, competitors, regulators and payer organisation; payer organisation can cause an extreme change in plans, from rapid acceleration to a complete halt of the programme. In addition, corporate philosophy and goals, as well as organisational structure, can also impact a development programme's strategy.

Competition, both internal and external, is a difficult factor to manage. Competition can take the form of internal competition between indications for a compound's resources, as well as between compounds which address the same family of indications. The CDP should outline how to address this.

The approach in this chapter naturally emphasises strategic goals based on commercial experience. These strategic goals reflect both common, clinical and scientific goals and relevant corporate financial opportunities and challenges, since maintaining positive cash flow, and the extent of that income source, will dictate potential opportunities and risks. For any publicly traded company, the value of the investigational portfolio is intrinsically incorporated into the value of the stock price. A failed phase III trial can strongly influence the stock price of a company if this compound reflects a sizable portion of the stock price as well as an erosion of confidence in the company to register drugs. Decisions which benefit the company are at the level of the clinical trial, such as minimising patients who are exposed to toxic drugs via careful sample size determination and interim analyses. Other decisions at the strategic level, including selection of drugs with most appropriate benefit/risk balance, and the efficient development of viable therapies also benefit both patients and society as a whole. While this could be done formally using a decision-theoretic framework, it is often informally managed.

13.3   Selecting designs by strategy

The CDP provides guidance in terms of overall goals and approaches for clinical development. Since it has a strategic focus for approaching clinical development, a selection of trial designs based on strategic deliverables is simpler for teams to use. We first give some examples of overall programme-level strategies that could be under consideration, before moving forward with how a few common phase II strategies are addressed.

Overall programme strategies are described differently from, and yet contain, the phase II strategies which are being considered. For example, one increasingly popular development strategy is to target a rare but well-characterised oncological indication, register the compound for treatment in that setting and then construct a series of interrelated development programmes to expand into different indications. These expanded indications are selected by considering the targets which represent a component of the tumour, unlike the original indication where the target is found more homogenously across the whole tumour. Another strategy is to leverage chemical synergies and initially target a medium-sized indication based on initial pre-clinical and phase I results, combined with how they may relate to existing medical practice and needs. Other common strategies include pairing new treatments with existing ones for combination therapies, as well as including in the initial plans a focus on setting up a possible diagnostic/compound combination.

Phase II studies address the middle stage of these strategies. For each example given above, multiple questions could be addressed depending on the specific tactical implementation of the global CDP strategy. The rest of this section focuses on the phase II-specific strategic aspects.

13.3.1   Basic strategies addressed by phase II studies

The summary within Table 13.1 illustrates some examples of matching trial design options to development strategies. For each strategy, multiple phase II designs are observed to have been employed, and some of these designs can be seen to have addressed multiple strategic objectives. This table is just a historical view; proper due diligence requires searching the literature for improvements and newer designs which may include any of those listed within Chapters 3–7, understanding available data in the specific setting and the current state of regulatory requirements and payer opinions. Based on an internal review of phase II experiences, we have identified six strategic goals that have occurred with high frequency, specifically:

1. Determination of activity for registration

2. Determine exploratory activity

3. Selection of regimen (single and combination agents)

4. Prediction of phase III success

5. Safety characterisation

6. Prospective identification of target populations

A clinical development programme can have multiple phase II trials, sometimes answering the same strategic question on a different topic (different safety foci, different subgroups to characterise). Alternatively, a single phase II trial can address multiple goals. We now cover each strategy and describe considerations as well as some of the trial design features which are of increasing importance for each particular strategy.

13.3.2   Potential registration

The first strategic goal discussed is the accommodation of possible registration based on strong positive early results. This could be considered a feasible strategic goal based on pre-clinical data, phase I study results and the overall scientific and medical rationale for development. The considerations in this section are primarily applicable to situations when conditional or accelerated approval is based solely on phase II or earlier trial data. Although this section primarily relates to trials designed for registration, it also applies to registration from trials in which overwhelming evidence of efficacy was observed although not planned for registration. Registration trials designed to meet the usual requirement of 'an adequate and well-controlled study' are out of scope for this section; for example, we do not cover intended phase III trials powered to detect clinically meaningful differences at the one-sided 2.5% level of significance.

13.3.2.1   Regulatory considerations

This strategic goal intersects regulatory and statistical considerations. It is critical to remember that the regulatory environment is constantly changing and requires

Table 13.1 Roadmap for phase II: strategic situations.

Known at phase II planning	Main goal of phase II study	Major designs	Major endpoints (most common)
Regimen likely to be active in an unmet medical need without approved or available therapy, no major safety issues	Determine potential for phase II-based registration (endpoint to confer clinical benefit)	**Single-stage** and two-stage single-arm design *Randomised phase II*	Overall tumour response rate (e.g. durable CR) PFS, OS (overwhelming evidence of efficacy)
Phase I data available, dose known but activity in indication to be shown, not suitable for phase II registration, no major safety issues	Determine biological activity using a quick, intermediate endpoint	**Two-stage design**, single arm (Simon and Bayesian based) **Randomised phase II** **Single-arm multinomial** *Randomised two-stage multinomial* *Randomised discontinuation* *Growth modulation index (GMI)* *(intra-patient PFS)*	Overall tumour response rate (CR/PR) PFS, tumour markers, imaging 'wet' biomarker Multinomial (CR/PR, SD, early PD) Duration of SD GMI response rate (GMI ≥ 1.33)
Several potential regimens (doses, schedules, formulations, etc.) for possible combination development	Determine best regimen (possibly a combination) for subsequent randomised controlled trial	**Randomised Simon two stage** Randomised selection (Bayesian and frequentist) with and without control group Randomised (combination add-on vs. SOC) ***Randomised modified factorial (no control group)*** Randomised factorial (add-on with SOC)	Overall tumour response rate PFS Possibly pharmacodynamics

(continued)

Table 13.1 (Continued)

Known at phase II planning	Main goal of phase II study	Major designs	Major endpoints (most common)
Regimen, indication known, important to reduce risk in phase III; not suitable for phase II registration, no major safety issues	Determine likelihood of success in phase III using suitable endpoint and patient population in phase II study	**Randomised phase II (Bayesian-based predictive probability of success)**	Phase III endpoints PFS, OS, response rates (haematological malignancies)
Potential major safety issue(s) representing possible 'no/go'	Better characterise safety profile, especially major safety issue(s), include safety as co-primary endpoint	**Extension of two-stage designs where safety and efficacy are co-primary endpoints** **Seamless phase I/II** **Randomised phase II**	Safety and efficacy (usually overall tumour response rate)
Regimen, indication known but not suitable for phase II registration, no major safety issues, heterogeneous populations defined by molecular markers, histology, prior treatment paradigms	Determine appropriate patient subpopulation for phase III trial	**Adaptive targeted two-stage design** **'Basket of indication' design** **Stratification and enrichment designs**	Overall tumour response rate PFS Pharmacodynamics

Entries given in Bold, used in Novartis trials, italics, used in other pharma, bold italics, academic trials or literature.

regular review during the overall clinical development process. For phase II trials designed for registration, it is even more critical to review the most current regulatory guidance and recent relevant regulatory events, and regulatory affairs specialists need to be involved in design discussions.

Although regulatory approval based solely on phase II data still remains possible in both the United States and European Union (EU), its applicability may now be confined to indications for which there is no approved or available therapy and will likely require demonstration of clear clinical benefit and efficacy. One necessary but not sufficient programme-related requirement is that the accelerated approval (phase II) trial must be part of a well-conceived and comprehensive CDP. This CDP should include at least two randomised phase III trials for the registered indication which are planned as part of a post-marketing approval requirement. These phase III trials should be enrolling patients at the time of accelerated approval. The conditional marketing authorisation approval process in the EU is analogous to accelerated approval in the United States. However, it must be renewed on an annual basis. This renewal requires timely completion of studies demonstrating clinical benefit. Health authority meetings should be planned to confirm the adequacy of the registration plan including post-marketing approval commitments. For example, registration using single-arm trials based on objective tumour response rate may require evidence of strong positive benefit/risk, require documentation of unmet medical need or represent a rare indication.

If the planned phase II study for monotherapy or combination studies is intended for potential registration, this should be confirmed with the health authorities prior to the start of the study, for example, at the end of a phase I meeting. The briefing documents should also contain a detailed description of the planned phase II trial (detailed protocol synopsis), an overall CDP which includes concrete and viable plans for post-approval confirmatory trial(s) and a discussion about the total number of patients in the proposed submission to monitor safety (i.e. the size of the safety database). At the present time, the protocol would need to be submitted for an FDA Special Protocol Assessment (SPA), with content of the briefing documents similar to those prepared to discuss phase II-based registration with the Committee for Medicinal Products for Human Use (CHMP). They should provide evidence that the planned development would meet the requisite statutory requirements for conditional approval or approval under exceptional circumstances. For a single-arm trial, the absolute minimum evidence could be, for example, clear documentation that the investigated indication represents an unmet medical need (e.g. documentation that patients had progressive disease under standard of care) or represents a rare indication for which a randomised controlled trial is not feasible. Clearly, more evidence will be warranted if there are questions from regulators or others who are weighing the quality of the evidence.

While it is possible for a randomised controlled phase II trial to demonstrate overwhelming evidence of efficacy, the standards are rather stringent (see Section 13.3.2.2). The screening randomised phase II trial should incorporate the same degree of rigour as the planned phase III trials. Ideally, it should use the same endpoint and patient population as the planned phase III trials.

13.3.2.2   Statistical considerations

The statistical considerations can be discussed in relation to the planned role of phase II in the development strategy, that is, whether the phase II trials are specifically targeted for accelerated approval and/or conditional registration.

Trials planned for registration (accelerated approval and/or conditional registration)   Regulatory and medical considerations generally drive the potential for accelerated registration. The study designs commonly considered arise from the unmet medical need/rare indication setting and include single-arm designs based on objective tumour response, randomised uncontrolled phase II trials (e.g. two different doses) and randomised controlled studies for rare diseases (if feasible). The single-arm design may have one stage (if early termination for lack of efficacy is not a concern because of phase I activity) or two stages (if early termination for futility is a requirement).

Although statistical methodology is used to design the pivotal phase II study, drive sample size considerations and provide operating characteristics, successful statistical results may only be necessary and not sufficient for health authority approval. In the uncontrolled setting, clinical considerations for the overall benefit/risk are critical considerations.

As the CHMP guidance (EMEA/357981/2005) stipulates, statistical support is required to provide justification for 'approval based on exceptional circumstances'. Some of this is used to characterise the context of the design and indication; for example, the sponsor's inability to provide comprehensive efficacy and safety information because the rarity of the indication must be established. Evaluation of sample size requirements under various statistical scenarios may prove necessary to support an exceptional circumstances claim. Relevant EMA guidance such as the CHMP guidance on small populations, and the EMA workshop on methodological aspects of clinical trials for efficacy evaluations in small populations, should be referenced for possible alternative designs.

Trials not planned for registration but overwhelming evidence of efficacy observed   In addition to phase II trials planned for registration, it may be possible for a randomised controlled phase II trial designed for screening agents for subsequent phase III studies to provide overwhelming evidence of efficacy that might lead to registration. For example, if the primary efficacy endpoint and patient population match what is planned for phase III, a strong positive outcome may render a subsequent randomised controlled trial difficult to recruit and potentially unethical. With respect to design characteristics, it has been suggested that the boundaries used for interim monitoring of a randomised phase III trial be employed to determine overwhelming evidence of efficacy from a randomised phase II trial. For example, if there are one-quarter the number of events in the randomised phase II trial as compared to a randomised phase III trial, then a one-sided p-value <0.00003 would be required to claim efficacy, assuming O'Brien–Fleming boundaries are used for interim monitoring at 25% of the information.

Implementation and design should address the exceptional circumstances upon which the argument for registration is based. The impact on trial operations based on different outcomes must be contemplated. The regulatory acceptance of a claim based on a randomised controlled phase II trial not primarily or originally intended for submission but in which overwhelming evidence of efficacy was observed might be enhanced by pre-specifying this in the protocol. In this situation, consider providing a potential strategy for confirming an effect and for generating adequate safety information.

13.3.3 Exploratory activity

The goal of exploratory activity trials (phase IIa) is to collect efficacy data to use in planning for (or against) future randomised controlled trials. The phase IIa criteria should be explicitly defined and reflect the competitive environment and the appropriate level of evidence to decide on the merits of a subsequent larger randomised controlled trial at a particular level of risk.

Risk calculations must, at least implicitly, incorporate expected returns. From a pharmaceutical company perspective, the cost of not continuing development of a 'good' drug, in terms of expected future sales, might be much greater than continuing with a bad drug. On one side, continuing development of a 'bad' drug results in losses from the failed phase III trial as well as the lost opportunity of reallocating resources for better drugs. On the other, potential profit from a new successful drug could outweigh the potential losses from continuing with a useless or harmful drug; this can encourage continuing development in the case of uncertainty.

If they exist, short-term endpoints which are well correlated with the primary endpoint for registration should be considered as discussed in Chapter 2. This is still true even if they are not causally related to the registration endpoint. This data can help support a no-go decision (termination of development for the specific indication). In addition, a successful phase IIa trial may use the results from these endpoints to reassess the proposed future trial designs within the CDP.

Both single-arm and randomised trial designs (especially for combination agents) may be used for phase IIa trials.

Bayesian and frequentist methods have been proposed for phase IIa trials. For frequentist designs, the power of the pre-specified success criteria is key, since a negative trial for the phase IIa endpoint may terminate an indication's development. As discussed above, the risks involved in termination of a development programme require careful consideration. A greater type I error rate, increasing the tolerance for allowing a poor development programme to continue, may be tolerated in this phase IIa setting. For example, one-sided type I error rates as high as 20% have been used for randomised phase IIa trials and one-sided type I error rates as high as 10% have been used for internal single-arm phase IIa trials.

Bayesian methods can incorporate relevant historical information in a straightforward manner if it exists (Neuenschwander et al. 2010). Attention and preparation should be given to prepare for concerns regarding the selection of historical data (prior sensitivity) and operating characteristics under different scenarios, as previously discussed in Chapter 2. However, reliable historical data for the phase IIa study might not be available. If the trial relies on a functional imaging or molecular biomarker or is limited to a targeted subpopulation, this information may not be available for the standard of care. In other settings where historical information for the phase IIa endpoint may be available, there may be concerns about inter-trial variability that would indicate the need for a randomised phase IIa trial. Historical information is not necessarily usable on a one-to-one substitution basis as a replacement for including a control (active or placebo) arm in the study. In particular, a phase IIa trial for a combination of a new drug added to a standard of care should be a randomised comparison with the standard of care alone. One advantage to the Bayesian analysis approach is that it can also provide estimates of the predictive probability of success (PoS) in later trials. For further discussion of PoS refer to section 13.3.5.

Finally, we reiterate that data on potential phase III endpoints to support future trial planning and programme-level decision-making should be collected even though a short-term endpoint was chosen to design the phase IIa trial.

13.3.4   Regimen selection

Selection of a regimen for single-agent therapies tends to follow two strategies. If there is sufficient evidence of activity in all proposed experimental regimens, a randomised selection design without a control group may be used. Selection designs try to determine the best regimen when several competing regimens are candidates for a subsequent randomised controlled trial to study only the best regimen. For example, there may be questions about the most appropriate dose, schedule, sequence and/or formulation to compare with the standard of care. This aims to have a high chance of selecting the best regimen (if it exists) for a subsequent randomised controlled trial without requiring additional subjects in a placebo arm for comparison. The other common design strategy is to incorporate historical or concurrent controls in a traditional comparison design, potentially with the facility to drop ineffective regimens early. Historical controls should be carefully considered for relevance, as temporal changes in standard of care could increase bias, variance or both. Concurrent controls may be required due to insufficient information on activity. Chapter 5 in this book summarises additional design possibilities.

If there is a marked difference in response based on dose or regimen, selection designs are straightforward for comparing regimes of a single compound. However, it can be a valuable tool to select across compounds at the same stage of development. In this instance, there are many challenges to implementing the first strategy within a company. In many pharmaceutical companies, project teams are usually set up to develop individual drugs or drugs from the same family. Successful implementation for cross-compound selection would require either close collaboration across teams or an integrated indication team approach to development. This also applies to the selection stage in the development of combination therapies

13.3.4.1   Adaptive designs and selection

Regimen selection during the phase II part of an adaptive phase II/III design is one of the common adaptations cited by the proponents of the design. There are many positive aspects for these designs which are found in the literature. To balance out that view, we point out that the greatest obstacles to implementation of such an adaptive phase II/III design are primarily logistic. For example, there must be adequate firewalls in place to keep the project team blinded to the phase II results, detailed pre-specified decision rules for selecting the best regimen to be chosen by an independent group, usually a data monitoring committee (DMC), and one or more meetings with the health authorities. The potential advantages from using an adaptive phase II/III design with regimen selection during the phase II part should be weighed against the intensive and time-consuming study start-up activities. There may also be increased monitoring, more complex randomisation and potential issues concerning operational bias. In addition, from a corporate perspective, the main decision-making is allocated to an external DMC which reduces the flexibility, in case of surprising internal or external results which result in requiring major trial changes. As a result phase II/III trials can have drawbacks when there is not so much existing knowledge about the drug, target population and indication.

13.3.4.2   Dose selection for combination therapies

Combination therapies require additional critical consideration. Different agents are often at different stages of development. Seldom do the agents have equal amounts of prior information from internal clinical studies.

The intentional drug–drug interaction leads to considering a few subsequent points. With respect to safety there may be a synergistic effect of the combination of drugs leading to a higher incidence of severe acute and delayed toxicity relative to the single-agent therapies, even if full doses were tolerable according to the individual phase I studies. In addition, identifying predictive biomarkers for patient stratification may be more challenging in the combination setting. For combinations where one or more agent has been approved, the selection of the approved agent as a component of the treatment should take into account the relative frequency of usage of this agent globally as well as the pre-clinical and phase I evidence supporting the usage of the combination with the investigational agent. For registration of a combination therapy of two or more investigational agents the contribution to efficacy of each component generally needs to be quantified to show evidence that any observed clinical benefit is not entirely attributable to only one of the two single agents. Contributions of the components might be demonstrated in phase II based on a surrogate or pharmacodynamic marker using a factorial design (U.S. Department of Health and Human Services 2013).

Regimen selection in the setting of combination therapies with two or more experiment compounds increases complexity. Three possible settings are (i) combination of an investigational agent(s) with a standard of care; (ii) combination of two (or more) investigational agents in an indication without a standard of care; and (iii) combination of two (or more) investigational agents compared to a standard of care. In all three settings we currently consider only randomised trial designs. Van Glabbeke et al. (2002) claimed that 'non-randomised Phase II studies of drug combinations are often meaningless, sometimes misleading'. They gave two examples where use of non-randomised phase II combination studies may have led to misleading development. The first was a study on dose-intensive chemotherapeutic regimens for intermediate- and/or high-grade non-Hodgkin's lymphoma. Here, five subsequent randomised trials versus a CHOP (or CHOP-like control) all showed no objective benefit but greater toxicity and toxic death rates relative to the standard arm. The second was an autologous bone marrow transplantation (BMT) for breast cancer. In this case, a definitive randomised phase III trial had accrual problems because of the reports of uncontrolled phase II trials.

13.3.5   Phase II to support predicting success in phase III

Predicting success in phase III is an important strategic consideration for the drug industry. In general, despite all of the introduced improvements in clinical development, the rate of phase III failures is still high, and it is common for management to be continually surprised by this. One of the reasons for this strategic goal is to manage expectations on what will be obtained from phase III trials, and therefore using previous data to predict the likelihood of 'success' is very appealing. If there is still a lot of uncertainty following phase II, then management must be aware of this so they can make appropriate planning decisions. At the end of the day companies can live with risk of 'failure' if it is well managed and spread appropriately across the portfolio.

Prospective thinking about the future success of a trial is an important part of good decision-making. Considerations of probability of success (PoS) comprise qualitative as well as quantitative aspects. There are various important qualitative considerations, such as the choice of endpoint, patient population, disease setting and dosing schedule. In order to be reasonably well calibrated, calculations of the PoS should include all relevant sources of uncertainty. These comprise uncertainties regarding the future data, the true underlying parameter of interest (e.g. a progression-free survival (PFS) hazard ratio), between-trial heterogeneity and the relationship between different endpoints in phases II and III.

From a predictive point of view, the most informative phase II design is a randomised design with the same endpoint (PFS or overall survival (OS)) as in phase III. For such a design, and a reasonably promising effect estimate in phase II (e.g. HR of 0.7 to 0.75), the PoS in phase III is approximately 60–70%. If a different endpoint is considered for phase II, collecting information on the phase III endpoint, if feasible, will be important. In summary,

- not acknowledging relevant uncertainties leads to an overly optimistic estimate for the PoS in phase III;

- the largest uncertainties should be accounted for since they have the largest impact;

- a good outcome in phase II does not necessarily lead to higher probabilities of success, in particular if between-trial heterogeneity is large.

A good quantitative estimate for the PoS is an important input for decision-making. For example, in a multi-stage trial this probability may inform decisions at interim to stop the trial early. Or, at the end of a phase II trial, the decision to go to phase III may be easier if the chance to be successful is reasonably high. However, formal quantifications of the PoS have not been used systematically in the past, for various reasons:

1. An assessment of the PoS in a future trial requires an understanding of future data, that is, a **prediction** for the data in the upcoming trial.

2. The inherent difficulty to make predictions. This is due to the fact that **extrapolations** are required from current data to future data, which are based on assumptions that are essentially unverifiable at the time when the prediction is made. The standard assumption is that the future will be identical to the past. To relax this fairly strong assumption means to introduce other assumptions that may be equally difficult to justify.

3. The need to think (before starting phase II) about the **design of the phase III trial**.

4. **Technical difficulties** that are of a purely statistical or computational nature.

Points 1 and 2 above are scientifically challenging. Predictions are one variant of the problem of induction (Hacking 2001), one of the most difficult problems in the empirical sciences. Predictions are inductive in the sense that there is no logical (or deductive) way that allows to reliably extrapolate (1) from partial to full information or (2) from the past to the future. The statistical/probabilistic approach to induction provides a quantitative framework that combines mathematical rigour with good judgement, the latter depending on the given context. To prospectively think about upcoming phase III trials, point 3, can be quite a challenge too, as it requires teams to think beyond phase II and may imply the involvement of health authorities at a fairly early stage.

Predictive problems in clinical trials arise in different ways:

1. The least controversial prediction problem is **within-trial prediction** for the same endpoint. This type of prediction may be of relevance at an interim stage of a phase IIa study. For example, in a multi-stage single-arm phase II trial, a prediction from the data on objective response rate (ORR) available at the first stage can be used to calculate the predictive distribution for the remaining data, from which the PoS for phase II can be obtained. This probability can be used to stop the trial, for futility and/or early success. Note that within-trial prediction is relatively straightforward only under the assumption that there is homogeneity over the different stages of the trial with regard to all relevant factors that may influence the outcome of the trial.

2. **Between-trial prediction** for the same endpoint is more difficult, because (in its simplest form) it critically depends on the assumption that all relevant factors that may influence the outcome are equal (or at least sufficiently similar) for both trials. For example, in a randomised phase II trial using a time-to-event

endpoint (e.g. a PFS hazard ratio), the data at the end of the trial can be used to predict data for an upcoming phase III trial of given design.

3. The quality of **between-endpoint prediction** depends on how predictive one endpoint is for the other. For example, PFS data may be collected in a randomised phase II trial, but OS will be used in phase III. Clearly, a proper prediction for PoS in phase III depends on a good understanding of the degree of correlation between PFS and OS. Therefore lack of knowledge between the endpoints adds to the uncertainty about the prediction and increases the challenges of planning across the portfolio, since risks of phase III failure are less known.

The different types of extrapolations may arise in combination. For example, in a phase II study with PFS as the primary endpoint, some limited information about OS may be available. For this situation, between-trial (for PFS) and between-trial as well as between-endpoint considerations (for OS) will influence the PoS in phase III. The level of uncertainty due to different endpoints depends also on the disease setting.

Prediction of future results in the context of clinical trials is an important use of early phase data and, as noted in this section, requires some attention to detail.

13.3.6   Phase II safety trials

Historically, within the drug industry, trials set up to specifically look at some aspect of safety have been relatively uncommon and have often been motivated as a result of health authority concerns. The evolving regulatory and reimbursement landscape has changed the playing field, and this drives development towards a situation where safety and specific risks are assessed in a proactive ongoing basis. It is assumed that the frequency of such studies will likely increase.

Although safety information is constantly monitored in all trials, sample size determination is usually based upon efficacy, and formal early stopping rules related to safety issues usually are not always clearly specified in phase II. Safety should be investigated as a co-primary endpoint when the study drug shows some preliminary efficacy but major safety concerns in the early stage of the development, or if the experimental treatment has similar efficacy as the standard but may have a substantial improvement of safety.

There are many advantages of collecting and studying safety data in phase II trials. For example, the safety data from phase II trials are collected in a more specific and controlled setting. Safety profiles in the targeted population(s) can provide further insight into the safety and efficacy relationship of the studied drug. Another example is that long-term toxicities or safety trends can be collected and studied. Phase I oncology trials usually have short duration and focus on the toxicities occurred in the first cycle in order to determine the maximum tolerated dose (MTD), and further recommended phase II dose. Finally, a control arm can be included to compare the safety profile of an investigational drug with the control of interest. Most of the time, the control could be a standard of care that is available to the general patient population.

The designs with both safety and efficacy as co-primary endpoints include, but are not limited to, Bryant and Day (1995), Conaway and Petroni (1995) and Thall and Cheng (2001) are discussed in more detail in Chapter 6. Additionally Hoering et al. (2011) consider this in the phase I/II setting. One practical problem with many of these designs is that defining toxicity as a binary variable can be clinically challenging when several toxicities of various grades are of interest.

13.3.7 Prospective identification of target populations

The increasing awareness that cancers are actually very heterogeneous has driven the development of targeted therapies which are effective in clearly defined and diagnosed populations. Although the number of potential patients may be reduced, this possible income loss can be balanced out by both a more powerful and stronger treatment effect (smaller and faster trials) and the likelihood of possible earlier approval where the additional time on the market can lead to increased income. A related challenge for pharmaceutical companies is that in many countries reimbursement must be justified, in that the payers require evidence for the population which will benefit most. Therefore, from a drug company point of view there is a financial imperative to ensure that the right set of patients are treated and that an appropriate level of evidence of efficacy is provided to the health authorities in this population.

Heterogeneity in treatment outcome is a common phenomenon in phase II clinical trials, perhaps more so than in phase III. Sources of heterogeneity of clinical outcome in response to an experimental treatment in phase II experiments can often be anticipated. The use of biomarkers can be one attempt to prospectively account for and control the variation. Without successful accommodation, the impact of unaccounted heterogeneity can lead to biased inferences. This can result in the early rejection of effective therapeutics or improper planning and failure in phase III experiments.

Two main design strategies, stratification and enrichment, are used (sometimes together) to prospectively account for such heterogeneity, as has previously been introduced in Chapter 2. First, enrichment strategies limit trial enrolment to patients with specific marker profiles. These should be used carefully and only in the presence of substantial contextual evidence that the study drug will be ineffective in the excluded patient subgroups. Second, stratification strategies enrol all comers but assess treatment effects separately in mutually exclusive subgroups. Such studies should be sized adequately to provide valid inferences about the effect (often benefit–risk) within each subgroup. For both of these approaches, adaptive and Bayesian variations of these strategies may be more informative and allow greater flexibility, although requiring considerable upfront investment for planning and implementation.

The choice of a phase II design depends on the nature of the marker(s) likely to affect treatment outcome in any given setting. Markers (single traits or signatures of traits) that are informative for clinical outcome can be broadly categorised as *predictive*, which are those that separate different populations in terms of the clinical outcome of interest in response to a particular treatment; or *prognostic*, those that separate different populations in terms of the clinical outcome of interest irrespective of the treatment; or *predictive–prognostic,* when both predictive and prognostic effects are observed.

Traditional approaches may be inadequate for a number of reasons. The main issue with traditional 'all-comers' designs is that they exercise no control on the subgroup composition of the set of patients studied. When the studied treatment is effective only in selected subgroups, the measured treatment effect is diluted and can lead to misleading conclusions and costly errors in development. This is particularly true for targeted agents.

For multiple reasons it is often not possible to retrospectively calculate accurate estimates of treatment effects within subgroups of interest (e.g. patients with a certain biomarker-positive status). Sample sizes of phase II cancer trials are often fairly small, so that there may be too few patients in a given subgroup (e.g. rare mutations) to draw reliable inference. Furthermore, without prospective planning important predictive traits may be confounded with other predictive/prognostic traits.

In comparative assessment of treatment benefit, randomisation can be used to achieve balance between treatment arms. However, in the case of predictive markers, without appropriate stratification there may still be important imbalances and confounding of effects due to small sample sizes, and the trial may therefore yield insufficient information to identify important subgroups.

For genetic and molecular markers, it is assumed that assays are available and have reasonable turnaround time to allow each patient's marker status to be established upfront (i.e. before enrolment or start of treatment). Definition of indications and hence designs for identifying indications are based on classification of biomarker status into a few discrete categories (typically a dichotomy). Thus, while biomarker status may be continuous, in most cases appropriate thresholds for classification need to be established prior to implementing the proposed strategies.

The relative merits of the proposed strategies need to be assessed at the outset and can be measured in terms of numbers of patients, time to completion of the trial or the cost of the trial. These merits are impacted by factors including the relative treatment effect in the biomarker-defined subgroups, the prevalence of these subgroups and the accuracy and cost of the diagnostic and treatment. Phase II designs which may be appropriate in the context of targeted subgroups are outlined in Chapter 7.

As a final note, when indications are based on levels of predictive biomarkers, co-development of reliable diagnostics for patient selection should start early. Failure to start early enough will increase risk due to the need to bridge between a clinical trial assay and a clinically and analytically validated diagnostic system.

13.4 Discussion

This chapter is intended to provide a strategic overview of programme-level decision-making and the need to tailor phase II designs according to the CDP. It is also intended to complement the other chapters in this book. By refining the strategic boundaries of what the trial should support, and then working to select the best of the implementable designs, this will result in more efficient trials which have a better chance to provide answers. Sometimes these trials will be shorter or smaller, but hopefully they will always be more decisive trials.

Phase II clinical trials play a critical role in understanding better how the compound can be used to maintain or improve the health of a patient. During times of rapid discovery of possible therapies, phase II trials can sometimes be viewed negatively, as an attempt to correct early mistaken decisions about the indicated use of the compound. During times when few compounds are being discovered, they can be seen as an opportunity and means to patiently increase the probability of finding a commercially viable and profitable niche for the compound. The challenge in understanding the huge diversity of designs, along with the ever-evolving commercial and medical landscape, makes the approach for proper selection interesting and difficult.

Disclaimer: The opinions expressed in this chapter are solely those of the authors and not necessarily those of Novartis. Novartis does not guarantee the accuracy or reliability of the information provided herein.

References

Adams, R.A., Meade, A.M., Seymour, M.T., Wilson, R.H., Madi, A., Fisher, D., Kenny, S.L., Kay, E., Hodgkinson, E., Pope, M., Rogers, P., Wasan, H., Falk, S., Gollins, S., Hickish, T., Bessell, E.M., Propper, D., Kennedy, M.J., Kaplan, R., Maughan, T.S. and MRC COIN Trial Investigators 2011. Intermittent versus continuous oxaliplatin and fluoropyrimidine combination chemotherapy for first-line treatment of advanced colorectal cancer: results of the randomised phase 3 MRC COIN Trial. *Lancet Oncology*, 12(7), 642–653.

Adjei, A.A., Christian, M. and Ivy, P. 2009. Novel designs and end points for phase II clinical trials. *Clinical Cancer Research*, 15(6), 1866–1872.

A'Hern, R.P. 2001. Sample size tables for exact single-stage phase II designs. *Statistics in Medicine*, 20(6), 859–866.

A'Hern, R.P. 2004. Widening eligibility to phase II trials: constant arcsine difference phase II trials. *Controlled Clinical Trials*, 25(3), 251–264.

An, M.W., Mandrekar, S.J. and Sargent, D.J. 2012. A 2-stage phase II design with direct assignment option in stage II for initial marker validation. *Clinical Cancer Research*, 18(16), 4225–4233.

Anderson, K.C., Kyle, R.A., Rajkumar, S.V., Stewart, A.K., Weber, D. and Richardson, P. 2007. Clinically relevant end points and new drug approvals for myeloma. *Leukemia*, 22(2), 231–239.

Anderson, K.C., Pazdur, R. and Farrell, A.T. 2005. Development of effective new treatments for multiple myeloma. *Journal of Clinical Oncology*, 23(28), 7207–7211.

Atkinson, A.J., Colburn, W.A., DeGruttola, V.G., DeMets, D.L., Downing, G.J., Hoth, D.F., Oates, J.A., Peck, C.C., Schooley, R.T., Spilker, B.A., Woodcock, J. and Zeger, S.L. 2001. Biomarkers and surrogate endpoints: preferred definitions and conceptual framework. *Clinincal Pharmacology and Therapeutics*, 69(3), 89–95.

Ayanlowo, A.O. and Redden, D.T. 2007. Stochastically curtailed phase II clinical trials. *Statistics in Medicine*, 26(7), 1462–1472.

Azzoli, C.G., Baker, S. Jr, Temin, S., Pao, W., Aliff, T., Brahmer, J., Johnson, D.H., Laskin, J.L., Masters, G., Milton, D., Nordquist, L., Pfister, D.G., Piantadosi, S., Schiller, J.H., Smith, R., Smith, T.J., Strawn, J.R., Trent, D., Giaccone, G. and American

Society of Clinical Oncology 2009. American Society of Clinical Oncology Clinical Practice Guideline update on chemotherapy for stage IV non-small-cell lung cancer. *Journal of Clinical Oncology*, 27(36), 6251–6266.

Banerjee, A. and Tsiatis, A.A. 2006. Adaptive two-stage designs in phase II clinical trials. *Statistics in Medicine*, 25(19), 3382–3395.

Bauer, M., Bauer, P. and Budde, M. 1998. A simulation program for adaptive two stage designs. *Computational Statistics & Data Analysis*, 26, 351–371.

Bauer, P. and Kieser, M. 1999. Combining different phases in the development of medical treatments within a single trial. *Statistics in Medicine*, 18(14), 1833–1848.

Bellissant, E., Benichou, J. and Chastang, C. 1990. Application of the triangular test to phase II cancer clinical trials. *Statistics in Medicine*, 9(8), 907–917.

Belvedere, O., Follador, A., Rossetto, C., Merlo, V., Defferrari, C., Sibau, A.M., Aita, M., Dal Bello, M.G., Meduri, S., Gaiardo, M., Fasola, G. and Grossi, F. 2011. A randomised phase II study of docetaxel/oxaliplatin and docetaxel in patients with previously treated non-small cell lung cancer: an Alpe-Adria Thoracic Oncology Multidisciplinary group trial (ATOM 019). *European Journal of Cancer*, 47(11), 1653–1659.

Bokemeyer, C., Bondarenko, I., Makhson, A., Hartmann, J.T., Aparicio, J., de Braud, F., Donea, S., Ludwig, H., Schuch, G., Stroh, C., Loos, A.H., Zubel, A. and Koralewski, P. 2009. Fluorouracil, leucovorin, and oxaliplatin with and without cetuximab in the first-line treatment of metastatic colorectal cancer. *Journal of Clinical Oncology*, 27(5), 663–671.

Booth, C.M., Calvert, A.H., Giaccone, G., Lobbezoo, M.W., Eisenhauer, E.A. and Seymour, L.K. 2008. Design and conduct of phase II studies of targeted anticancer therapy: recommendations from the task force on methodology for the development of innovative cancer therapies (MDICT). *European Journal of Cancer*, 44(1), 25–29.

Bretz, F., Schmidli, H., Konig, F., Racine, A. and Maurer, W. 2006. Confirmatory seamless phase II/III clinical trials with hypotheses selection at interim: general concepts. *Biometrical Journal*, 48(4), 623–634.

Brown, S.R., Gregory, W.M., Twelves, C.J., Buyse, M., Collinson, F., Parmar, M., Seymour, M.T. and Brown, J.M. 2011. Designing phase II trials in cancer: a systematic review and guidance. *British Journal of Cancer*, 105(2), 194–199.

Bryant, J. and Day, R. 1995. Incorporating toxicity considerations into the design of two-stage phase II clinical trials. *Biometrics*, 51(4), 1372–1383.

Burzykowski, T., Buyse, M., Piccart-Gebhart, M.J., Sledge, G., Carmichael, J., Luck, H.J., Mackey, J.R., Nabholtz, J.M., Paridaens, R., Biganzoli, L., Jassem, J., Bontenbal, M., Bonneterre, J., Chan, S., Basaran, G.A. and Therasse, P. 2008. Evaluation of tumor response, disease control, progression-free survival, and time to progression as potential surrogate end points in metastatic breast cancer. *Journal of Clinical Oncology*, 26(12), 1987–1992.

Buyse, M. 2000. Randomized designs for early trials of new cancer treatments – an overview. *Drug Information Journal*, 34(2) 387–396.

Buyse, M., Burzykowski, T., Carroll, K., Michiels, S., Sargent, D.J., Miller, L.L., Elfring, G.L., Pignon, J.P. and Piedbois, P. 2007. Progression-free survival is a surrogate for survival in advanced colorectal cancer. *Journal of Clinical Oncology*, 25(33), 5218–5224.

Buyse, M., Michiels, S., Sargent, D.J., Grothey, A., Matheson, A. and de Gramont, A. 2011. Integrating biomarkers in clinical trials. *Expert Review of Molecular Diagnostics*, 11(2), 171–182.

Buyse, M., Molenberghs, G., Burzykowski, T., Renard, D. and Geys, H. 2000. The validation of surrogate endpoints in meta-analyses of randomized experiments. *Biostatistics*, 1(1), 49–67.

Cannistra, S.A. 2009. Phase II trials in Journal of Clinical Oncology. *Journal of Clinical Oncology*, 27(19), 3073–3076.

Capra, W.B. 2004. Comparing the power of the discontinuation design to that of the classic randomized design on time-to-event endpoints. *Controlled Clinical Trials*, 25(2), 168–177.

Case, L.D. and Morgan, T.M. 2003. Design of phase II cancer trials evaluating survival probabilities. *BMC Medical Research Methodology*, 3, 1–12.

Chang, M.N., Devidas, M. and Anderson, J. 2007. One- and two-stage designs for phase II window studies. *Statistics in Medicine*, 26(13), 2604–2614.

Chang, M.N., Shuster, J.J. and Kepner, J.L. 1999. Group sequential designs for phase II trials with historical controls. *Controlled Clinical Trials*, 20(4), 353–364.

Chang, M.N., Shuster, J.J. and Kepner, J.L. 2004. Sample sizes based on exact unconditional tests for phase II clinical trials with historical controls. *Journal of Biopharmaceutical Statistics*, 14(1), 189–200.

Chang, M.N., Therneau, T.M., Wieand, H.S. and Cha, S.S. 1987. Designs for group sequential phase II clinical trials. *Biometrics*, 43(4), 865–874.

Chen, C. and Beckman, R.A. 2009. Optimal cost-effective designs of phase II proof of concept trials and associated go-no go decisions. *Journal of Biopharmaceutical Statistics*, 19(3), 424–436.

Chen, C. and Chaloner, K. 2006. A Bayesian stopping rule for a single arm study: with a case study of stem cell transplantation. *Statistics in Medicine*, 25(17), 2956–2966.

Chen, K. and Shan, M. 2008. Optimal and minimax three-stage designs for phase II oncology clinical trials. *Contemporary Clinical Trials*, 29(1), 32–41.

Chen, S., Soong, S.J. and Wheeler, R.H. 1994. An efficient multiple-stage procedure for phase II clinical trials that have high response rate objectives. *Controlled Clinical Trials*, 15(4), 277–283.

Chen, T.T. 1997. Optimal three-stage designs for phase II cancer clinical trials. *Statistics in Medicine*, 16(23), 2701–2711.

Chen, T.T. and Ng, T.H. 1998. Optimal flexible designs in phase II clinical trials. *Statistics in Medicine*, 17(20), 2301–2312.

Cheung, Y.K. 2009. Selecting promising treatments in randomized phase II cancer trials with an active control. *Journal of Biopharmaceutical Statistics*, 19(3), 494–508.

Cheung, Y.K. and Thall, P.F. 2002. Monitoring the rates of composite events with censored data in phase II clinical trials. *Biometrics*, 58(1), 89–97.

Chi, Y. and Chen, C.M. 2008. Curtailed two-stage designs in phase II clinical trials. *Statistics in Medicine*, 27(29), 6175–6189.

Chow, S.C. and Tu, Y.H. 2008. On two-stage seamless adaptive design in clinical trials. *Journal of the Formosan Medical Association*, 107(Suppl 12), 52–60.

Collette, L., Burzykowski, T., Carroll, K.J., Newling, D., Morris, T. and Schroder, F.H. 2005. Is prostate-specific antigen a valid surrogate end point for survival in hormonally treated patients with metastatic prostate cancer? Joint Research of the European Organisation for Research and Treatment of Cancer, the Limburgs Universitair Centrum, and AstraZeneca Pharmaceuticals. *Journal of Clinical Oncology*, 23(25), 6139–6148.

Collier, R. 2009. Drug development cost estimates hard to swallow. *Canadian Medical Association Journal*, 180(3), 279–280.

Committee for Medicinal Products for Human Use (CHMP) 2005. *Guideline on Procedures for the Granting of a Marketing Authorisation Under Exceptional Circumstances, pursuant to Article 14 (8) of Regulation (EC) NO 726/2004 (EMEA/357981/2005)*.

Conaway, M.R. and Petroni, G.R. 1995. Bivariate sequential designs for phase II trials. *Biometrics*, 51(2), 656–664.

Conaway, M.R. and Petroni, G.R. 1996. Designs for phase II trials allowing for a trade-off between response and toxicity. *Biometrics*, 52(4), 1375–1386.

Cronin, K.A., Freedman, L.S., Lieberman, R., Weiss, H.L., Beenken, S.W. and Kelloff, G.J. 1999. Bayesian monitoring of phase II trials in cancer chemoprevention. *Journal of Clinical Epidemiology*, 52(8), 705–711.

de Boo, T.M. and Zielhuis, G.A. 2004. Minimization of sample size when comparing two small probabilities in a non-inferiority safety trial. *Statistics in Medicine*, 23(11), 1683–1699.

Dhani, N., Tu, D., Sargent, D.J., Seymour, L. and Moore, M.J. 2009. Alternate endpoints for screening phase II studies. *Clinical Cancer Research*, 15(6), 1873–1882.

DiMasi, J.A. and Grabowski, H.G. 2007. Economics of new oncology drug development. *Journal of Clinical Oncology*, 25(2), 209–216.

Eisenhauer, E.A., Therasse, P., Bogaerts, J., Schwartz, L.H., Sargent, D., Ford, R., Dancey, J., Arbuck, S., Gwyther, S., Mooney, M., Rubinstein, L., Shankar, L., Dodd, L., Kaplan, R., Lacombe, D. and Verweij, J. 2009. New response evaluation criteria in solid tumours: revised RECIST guideline (version 1.1). *European Journal of Cancer*, 45(2), 228–247.

Ensign, L.G., Gehan, E.A., Kamen, D.S. and Thall, P.F. 1994. An optimal three-stage design for phase II clinical trials. *Statistics in Medicine*, 13(17), 1727–1736.

Facon, T., Mary, J.Y., Hulin, C., Benboubker, L., Attal, M., Pegourie, B., Renaud, M., Harousseau, J.L., Guillerm, G., Chaleteix, C., Dib, M., Voillat, L., Maisonneuve, H., Troncy, J., Dorvaux, V., Monconduit, M., Martin, C., Casassus, P., Jaubert, J., Jardel, H., Doyen, C., Kolb, B., Anglaret, B., Grosbois, B., Yakoub-Agha, I., Mathiot, C., Avet-Loiseau, H. and Intergroupe Francophone du Myélome 2007. Melphalan and prednisone plus thalidomide versus melphalan and prednisone alone or reduced-intensity autologous stem cell transplantation in elderly patients with multiple myeloma (IFM 99-06): a randomised trial. *Lancet*, 370(9594), 1209–1218.

Fazzari, M., Heller, G. and Scher, H.I. 2000. The phase II/III transition. Toward the proof of efficacy in cancer clinical trials. *Controlled Clinical Trials*, 21(4), 360–368.

Fisher, R.A. 1932. *Statistical Methods for Research Workers*, 4th edn. Oliver and Boyd, Edinburgh.

Fleming, T.R. 1982. One-sample multiple testing procedure for phase II clinical trials. *Biometrics*, 38, 143–151.

Fossella, F.V., DeVore, R., Kerr, R.N., Crawford, J., Natale, R.R., Dunphy, F., Kalman, L., Miller, V., Lee, J.S., Moore, M., Gandara, D., Karp, D., Vokes, E., Kris, M., Kim, Y., Gamza, F. and Hammershaimb, L. 2000. Randomized phase III trial of docetaxel versus vinorelbine or ifosfamide in patients with advanced non-small-cell lung cancer previously treated with platinum-containing chemotherapy regimens. The TAX 320 Non-Small Cell Lung Cancer Study Group. [Erratum appears in *Journal of Clinical Oncology* 2004;22(1), 209]. *Journal of Clinical Oncology*, 18(12), 2354–2362.

Freedland, S.J., Humphreys, E.B. and Mangold, L.A. 2005. Risk of prostate cancer-specific mortality following biochemical recurrence after radical prostatectomy. *Journal of American Medical Association*, 294(4), 433–439.

Freidlin, B., Dancey, J., Korn, E.L., Zee, B. and Eisenhauer, E. 2002. Multinomial phase II trial designs. *Journal of Clinical Oncology*, 20(2), 599.

Freidlin, B. and Korn, E.L. 2013. Borrowing information across subgroups in phase II trials: is it useful? *Clinical Cancer Research*, 19(6), 1326–1334.

Freidlin, B., McShane, L.M., Polley, M.Y. and Korn, E.L. 2012. Randomized phase II trial designs with biomarkers. *Journal of Clinical Oncology*, 30(26), 3304–3309.

Freidlin, B. and Simon, R. 2005. Evaluation of randomized discontinuation design. *Journal of Clinical Oncology*, 23(22), 5094–5098.

Gajewski, B.J. and Mayo, M.S. 2006. Bayesian sample size calculations in phase II clinical trials using a mixture of informative priors. *Statistics in Medicine*, 25(15), 2554–2566.

Gehan, E.A. 1961. The determination of the number of patients required in a preliminary and a follow-up trial of a new chemotherapeutic agent. *Journal of Chronic Diseases*, 13(4), 346–353.

Giaccone, G., Herbst, R.S., Manegold, C., Scagliotti, G., Rosell, R., Miller, V., Natale, R.B., Schiller, J.H., von Pawel, J., Pluzanska, A., Gatzemeier, U., Grous, J., Ochs, J.S., Averbuch, S.D., Wolf, M.K., Rennie, P., Fandi, A. and Johnson, D.H. 2004. Gefitinib in combination with gemcitabine and cisplatin in advanced non-small-cell lung cancer: a phase III trial – INTACT 1. *Journal of Clinical Oncology*, 22(5), 777–784.

Goffin, J.R. and Tu, D. 2008. Phase II stopping rules that employ response rates and early progression. *Journal of Clinical Oncology*, 26(22), 3715–3720.

Goldman, A.I. 1987. Issues in designing sequential stopping rules for monitoring side effects in clinical trials. *Controlled Clinical Trials*, 8, 327–337.

Goldman, A.I. and Hannan, P.J. 2001. Optimal continuous sequential boundaries for monitoring toxicity in clinical trials: a restricted search algorithm. *Statistics in Medicine*, 20(11), 1575–1589.

Green, S.J. and Dahlberg, S. 1992. Planned versus attained design in phase II clinical trials. *Statistics in Medicine*, 11(7), 853–862.

Hacking, I. 2001. *An Introduction to Probability and Inductive Logic*. Cambridge University Press.

Hanfelt, J.J., Slack, R.S. and Gehan, E.A. 1999. A modification of Simon's optimal design for phase II trials when the criterion is median sample size. *Controlled Clinical Trials*, 20(6), 555–566.

Hanna, N., Shepherd, F.A., Fossella, F.V., Pereira, J.R., De Marinis, F., von Pawel, J., Gatzemeier, U., Tsao, T.C., Pless, M., Muller, T., Lim, H.L., Desch, C., Szondy, K., Gervais, R., Shaharyar, Manegold, C., Paul, S., Paoletti, P., Einhorn, L. and Bunn, P.A., Jr 2004. Randomized phase III trial of pemetrexed versus docetaxel in patients with non-small-cell lung cancer previously treated with chemotherapy. *Journal of Clinical Oncology*, 22(9), 1589–1597.

Heitjan, D.F. 1997. Bayesian interim analysis of phase II cancer clinical trials. *Statistics in Medicine*, 16(16), 1791–1802.

Herbst, R.S., Giaccone, G., Schiller, J.H., Natale, R.B., Miller, V., Manegold, C., Scagliotti, G., Rosell, R., Oliff, I., Reeves, J.A., Wolf, M.K., Krebs, A.D., Averbuch, S.D., Ochs, J.S., Grous, J., Fandi, A. and Johnson, D.H. 2004. Gefitinib in combination with paclitaxel and carboplatin in advanced non-small-cell lung cancer: a phase III trial – INTACT 2. *Journal of Clinical Oncology*, 22(5), 785–794.

Herndon, J.E. 1998. A design alternative for two-stage, phase II, multicenter cancer clinical trials. *Controlled Clinical Trials*, 19(5), 440–450.

Herson, J. 1979. Predictive probability early termination plans for phase II clinical trials. *Biometrics*, 35(4), 775–783.

Herson, J. and Carter, S.K. 1986. Calibrated phase II clinical trials in oncology. *Statistics in Medicine*, 5(5), 441–447.

Hoering, A., Leblanc, M. and Crowley, J. 2011. Seamless phase I–II trial design for assessing toxicity and efficacy for targeted agents. *Clinical Cancer Research*, 17(4), 640–646.

Hong, S. and Wang, Y. 2007. A three-outcome design for randomized comparative phase II clinical trials. *Statistics in Medicine*, 26(19), 3525–3534.

ICH Expert Working Group 1994. *International Conference on Harmonisation, Guideline on Dose-Response Information to Support Drug Registration E4.*

ICH Expert Working Group 1997. *International Conference on Harmonisation, Guideline on General Considerations for Clinical Trials E8.*

Ivanova, A., Qaqish, B.F. and Schell, M.J. 2005. Continuous toxicity monitoring in phase II trials in oncology. *Biometrics*, 61(2), 540–545.

Jenkins, M., Stone, A. and Jennison, C. 2011. An adaptive seamless phase II/III design for oncology trials with subpopulation selection using correlated survival endpoints. *Pharmaceutical Statistics*, 10(4), 347–356.

Jin, H. 2007. Alternative designs of phase II trials considering response and toxicity. *Contemporary Clinical Trials*, 28(4), 525–531.

Johnson, V.E. and Cook, J.D. 2009. Bayesian design of single-arm phase II clinical trials with continuous monitoring. *Clinical Trials*, 6(3), 217–226.

Jones, C.L. and Holmgren, E. 2007. An adaptive Simon two-stage design for phase 2 studies of targeted therapies. *Contemporary Clinical Trials*, 28(5), 654–661.

Jung, S.H. 2008. Randomized phase II trials with a prospective control. *Statistics in Medicine*, 27(4), 568–583.

Jung, S.H. and George, S.L. 2009. Between-arm comparisons in randomized phase II trials. *Journal of Biopharmaceutical Statistics*, 19(3), 456–468.

Jung, S.H., Lee, T., Kim, K. and George, S.L. 2004. Admissible two-stage designs for phase II cancer clinical trials. *Statistics in Medicine*, 23(4), 561–569.

Karrison, T.G., Maitland, M.L., Stadler, W.M. and Ratain, M.J. 2007. Design of phase II cancer trials using a continuous endpoint of change in tumor size: application to a study of sorafenib and erlotinib in non small-cell lung cancer. *Journal of the National Cancer Institute*, 99(19), 1455–1461.

Kelly, P.J., Stallard, N. and Todd, S. 2005. An adaptive group sequential design for phase II/III clinical trials that select a single treatment from several. *Journal of Biopharmaceutical Statistics*, 15(4), 641–658.

Kocherginsky, M., Cohen, E.E. and Karrison, T. 2009. Design of phase II cancer trials for evaluation of cytostatic/cytotoxic agents. *Journal of Biopharmaceutical Statistics*, 19(3), 524–529.

Kopec, J.A., Abrahamowicz, M. and Esdaile, J.M. 1993. Randomized discontinuation trials: utility and efficiency. *Journal of Clinical Epidemiology*, 46(9), 959–971.

Korn, E.L., Liu, P.Y., Lee, S.J., Chapman, J.A., Niedzwiecki, D., Suman, V.J., Moon, J., Sondak, V.K., Atkins, M.B., Eisenhauer, E.A., Parulekar, W., Markovic, S.N., Saxman, S. and Kirkwood, J.M. 2008. Meta-analysis of phase II cooperative group trials in metastatic stage IV melanoma to determine progression-free and overall survival benchmarks for future phase II trials. *Journal of Clinical Oncology*, 26(4), 527–534.

Koyama, T. and Chen, H. 2008. Proper inference from Simon's two-stage designs. *Statistics in Medicine*, 27(16), 3145–3154.

Lachin, J.M. and Younes, N. 2007. A composite design for transition from a preliminary to a full-scale study. *Statistics in Medicine*, 26(27), 5014–5032.

Lai, T.L., Lavori, P.W., Shih, M.C. and Sikic, B.I. 2012. Clinical trial designs for testing biomarker-based personalized therapies. *Clinical Trials*, 9(2), 141–154.

Le Blanc, M., Rankin, C. and Crowley, J. 2009. Multiple histology phase II trials. *Clinical Cancer Research*, 15(13), 4256–4262.

Lee, J.J. and Feng, L. 2005. Randomized phase II designs in cancer clinical trials: current status and future directions. *Journal of Clinical Oncology*, 23(19), 4450–4457.

Lee, J.J. and Liu, D.D. 2008. A predictive probability design for phase II cancer clinical trials. *Clinical Trials*, 5(2), 93–106.

Lee, Y.J., Staquet, M., Simon, R., Catane, R. and Muggia, F. 1979. Two-stage plans for patient accrual in phase II cancer clinical trials. *Cancer Treatment Reports*, 63(11–12), 1721–1726.

Levy, G., Kaufmann, P., Buchsbaum, R., Montes, J., Barsdorf, A., Arbing, R., Battista, V., Zhou, X., Mitsumoto, H., Levin, B. and Thompson, J.L. 2006. A two-stage design for a phase II clinical trial of coenzyme Q10 in ALS. *Neurology*, 66(5), 660–663.

Lin, D.Y., Shen, L., Ying, Z. and Breslow, N.E. 1996. Group sequential designs for monitoring survival probabilities. *Biometrics*, 52(3), 1033–1041.

Lin, S.P. and Chen, T.T. 2000. Optimal two-stage designs for phase II clinical trials with differentiation of complete and partial responses. *Communications in Statistics-Theory and Methods*, 29(5–6), 923–940.

Lin, Y. and Shih, W.J. 2004. Adaptive two-stage designs for single-arm phase IIA cancer clinical trials. *Biometrics*, 60(2), 482–490.

Litwin, S., Wong, Y.N. and Hudes, G. 2007. Early stopping designs based on progression-free survival at an early time point in the initial cohort. *Statistics in Medicine*, 26(24), 4400–4415.

Liu, Q. and Pledger, G.W. 2005. Phase 2 and 3 combination designs to accelerate drug development. *Journal of the American Statistical Association*, 100(470), 493–502.

Logan, B.R. 2005. Optimal two-stage randomized phase II clinical trials. *Clinical Trials*, 2(1), 5–12.

London, W.B. and Chang, M.N. 2005. One- and two-stage designs for stratified phase II clinical trials. *Statistics in Medicine*, 24(17), 2597–2611.

Lu, Y., Jin, H. and Lamborn, K.R. 2005. A design of phase II cancer trials using total and complete response endpoints. *Statistics in Medicine*, 24(20), 3155–3170.

Machin, D. and Campbell, M.J. 2005. *Design of Studies for Medical Research*. John Wiley & Sons, Ltd, Chichester.

Machin, D., Campbell, M.J., Tan, S.-B. and Tan, S.-H. 2008. *Sample Size Tables for Clinical Studies*, 3rd edn. Wiley-Blackwell.

Mandrekar, S.J., An, M.W. and Sargent, D.J. 2013. A review of phase II trial designs for initial marker validation. *Contemporary Clinical Trials,* Epub ahead of print.

Mandrekar, S.J., Qi, Y., Hillman, S.L., Allen Ziegler, K.L., Reuter, N.F., Rowland, K.M., Jr, Kuross, S.A., Marks, R.S., Schild, S.E. and Adjei, A.A. 2010. Endpoints in phase II trials for advanced non-small cell lung cancer. *Journal of Thoracic Oncology,* 5(1), 3–9.

Mariani, L. and Marubini, E. 1996. Design and analysis of phase II cancer trials: a review of statistical methods and guidelines for medical researchers. *International Statistical Review,* 64(1), 61–88.

Mariani, L. and Marubini, E. 2000. Content and quality of currently published phase II cancer trials. *Journal of Clinical Oncology,* 18(2), 429–436.

Mayo, M.S. and Gajewski, B.J. 2004. Bayesian sample size calculations in phase II clinical trials using informative conjugate priors. *Controlled Clinical Trials,* 25(2), 157–167.

McShane, L.M., Hunsberger, S. and Adjei, A.A. 2009. Effective incorporation of biomarkers into phase II trials. *Clinical Cancer Research,* 15(6), 1898–1905.

Michiels, S., Le Maitre, A., Buyse, M., Burzykowski, T., Maillard, E., Bogaerts, J., Vermorken, J.B., Budach, W., Pajak, T.F., Ang, K.K., Bourhis, J. and Pignon, J.P. 2009. Surrogate endpoints for overall survival in locally advanced head and neck cancer: meta-analyses of individual patient data. *The Lancet Oncology,* 10(4), 341–350.

Mick, R., Crowley, J.J. and Carroll, R.J. 2000. Phase II clinical trial design for noncytotoxic anticancer agents for which time to disease progression is the primary endpoint. *Controlled Clinical Trials,* 21(4), 343–359.

Monnet, I., Brienza, S., Hugret, F., Voisin, S., Gastiaburu, J., Saltiel, J.C., Soulie, P., Armand, J.P., Cvitkovic, E. and de Cremoux, H. 1998. Phase II study of oxaliplatin in poor-prognosis non-small cell lung cancer (NSCLC). ATTIT. Association pour le Traitement des Tumeurs Intra Thoraciques. *European Journal of Cancer,* 34(7), 1124–1127.

Murray, S.C., Otterness, M.F., Forster, J.K., Catellier, D.J. and Koch, G.G. 2004. An application of a multi-stage strategy involving confidence intervals to evaluate whether a response rate is favourable or not. *Pharmaceutical Statistics,* 3(1), 25–37.

Neuenschwander, B., Capkun-Niggli, G., Branson, M. and Spiegelhalter, D.J. 2010. Summarizing historical information on controls in clinical trials. *Clinical Trials,* 7(1), 5–18.

Norton, L. 2001. Theoretical concepts and the emerging role of taxanes in adjuvant therapy. *The Oncologist,* 6(Suppl 3), 30–35.

Norton, L. and Simon, R. 1977. Tumor size, sensitivity to therapy, and design of treatment schedules. *Cancer Treatment Reports,* 61(7), 1307–1317.

O'Brien, P.C. and Fleming, T.R. 1979. A multiple testing procedure for clinical trials. *Biometrics,* 35(3), 549–556.

Palumbo, A., Bringhen, S., Caravita, T., Merla, E., Capparella, V., Callea, V., Cangialosi, C., Grasso, M., Rossini, F., Galli, M., Catalano, L., Zamagni, E., Petrucci, M.T., De Stefano, V., Ceccarelli, M., Ambrosini, M.T., Avonto, I., Falco, P., Ciccone, G., Liberati, A.M., Musto, P., Boccadoro, M. and Italian Multiple Myeloma Network, GIMEMA. 2006. Oral melphalan and prednisone chemotherapy plus thalidomide compared with melphalan and prednisone alone in elderly patients with multiple myeloma: randomised controlled trial. *Lancet,* 367(9513), 825–831.

Palumbo, A., Bringhen, S., Liberati, A.M., Caravita, T., Falcone, A., Callea, V., Montanaro, M., Ria, R., Capaldi, A., Zambello, R., Benevolo, G., Derudas, D., Dore, F., Cavallo, F., Gay, F., Falco, P., Ciccone, G., Musto, P., Cavo, M. and Boccadoro, M. 2008. Oral melphalan, prednisone, and thalidomide in elderly patients with multiple myeloma: updated results of a randomized controlled trial. *Blood*, 112(8), 3107–3114.

Panageas, K.S., Smith, A., Gonen, M. and Chapman, P.B. 2002. An optimal two-stage phase II design utilizing complete and partial response information separately. *Controlled Clinical Trials*, 23(4), 367–379.

Pazdur, R. 2008. Endpoints for assessing drug activity in clinical trials. *The Oncologist*, 13(Suppl 2), 19–21.

Perrone, F., Di Maio, M., De Maio, E., Maione, P., Ottaiano, A., Pensabene, M., Di Lorenzo, G., Lombardi, A.V., Signoriello, G. and Gallo, C. 2003. Statistical design in phase II clinical trials and its application in breast cancer. *The Lancet Oncology*, 4(5), 305–311.

Piccart-Gebhart, M.J., Procter, M., Leyland-Jones, B., Goldhirsch, A., Untch, M., Smith, I., Gianni, L., Baselga, J., Bell, R., Jackisch, C., Cameron, D., Dowsett, M., Barrios, C.H., Steger, G., Huang, C.S., Andersson, M., Inbar, M., Lichinitser, M., Lang, I., Nitz, U., Iwata, H., Thomssen, C., Lohrisch, C., Suter, T.M., Ruschoff, J., Suto, T., Greatorex, V., Ward, C., Straehle, C., McFadden, E., Dolci, M.S. and Gelber, R.D. 2005. Trastuzumab after adjuvant chemotherapy in HER2-positive breast cancer. *New England Journal of Medicine*, 353(16), 1659–1672.

Piedbois, P. and Buyse, M. 2008. Endpoints and surrogate endpoints in colorectal cancer: a review of recent developments. *Current Opinion in Oncology*, 20(4), 466–471.

Pocock, S.J. 1977. Group sequential methods in the design and analysis of clinical trials. *Biometrika*, 64(2), 191–199.

Pound, C.R., Partin, A.W., Eisenberger, M.A., Chan, D.W., Pearson, J.D. and Walsh, P.C. 1999. Natural history of progression after PSA elevation following radical prostatectomy. *Journal of American Medical Association*, 281(17), 1591–1597.

Pusztai, L., Anderson, K. and Hess, K.R. 2007. Pharmacogenomic predictor discovery in phase II clinical trials for breast cancer. *Clinical Cancer Research*, 13(20), 6080–6086.

Redman, M. and Crowley, J. 2007. Small randomized trials. *Journal of Thoracic Oncology*, 2(1), 1–2.

Roberts, J.D. and Ramakrishnan, V. 2011. Phase II trials powered to detect tumor subtypes. *Clinical Cancer Research*, 17(17), 5538–5545.

Rosner, G.L., Stadler, W. and Ratain, M.J. 2002. Randomized discontinuation design: application to cytostatic antineoplastic agents. *Journal of Clinical Oncology*, 20(22), 4478–4484.

Royston, P., Parmar, M.K. and Qian, W. 2003. Novel designs for multi-arm clinical trials with survival outcomes with an application in ovarian cancer. *Statistics in Medicine*, 22(14), 2239–2256.

Rubinstein, L., Crowley, J., Ivy, P., Leblanc, M. and Sargent, D. 2009. Randomized phase II designs. *Clinical Cancer Research*, 15(6), 1883–1890.

Sambucini, V. 2008. A Bayesian predictive two-stage design for phase II clinical trials. *Statistics in Medicine*, 27(8), 1199–1224.

Sargent, D.J., Chan, V. and Goldberg, R.M. 2001. A three-outcome design for phase II clinical trials. *Controlled Clinical Trials*, 22(2), 117–125.

Sargent, D.J. and Goldberg, R.M. 2001. A flexible design for multiple armed screening trials. *Statistics in Medicine*, 20(7), 1051–1060.

Seymour, L., Ivy, S.P., Sargent, D., Spriggs, D., Baker, L., Rubinstein, L., Ratain, M.J., Le Blanc, M., Stewart, D., Crowley, J., Groshen, S., Humphrey, J.S., West, P. and Berry, D. 2010. The design of phase II clinical trials testing cancer therapeutics: consensus recommendations from the Clinical Trial Design Task Force of the National Cancer Institute Investigational Drug Steering Committee. *Clinical Cancer Research*, 16(6), 1764–1769.

Shepherd, F.A., Dancey, J., Ramlau, R., Mattson, K., Gralla, R., O'Rourke, M., Levitan, N., Gressot, L., Vincent, M., Burkes, R., Coughlin, S., Kim, Y. and Berille, J. 2000. Prospective randomized trial of docetaxel versus best supportive care in patients with non-small-cell lung cancer previously treated with platinum-based chemotherapy. *Journal of Clinical Oncology*, 18(10), 2095–2103.

Shun, Z., Lan, K.K. and Soo, Y. 2008. Interim treatment selection using the normal approximation approach in clinical trials. *Statistics in Medicine*, 27(4), 597–618.

Shuster, J. 2002. Optimal two-stage designs for single arm phase II cancer trials. *Journal of Biopharmaceutical Statistics*, 12(1), 39–51.

Simon, R. 1987. How large should a phase II trial of a new drug be? *Cancer Treatment Reports*, 71(11), 1079–1085.

Simon, R. 1989. Optimal two-stage designs for phase II clinical trials. *Controlled Clinical Trials*, 10(1), 1–10.

Simon, R., Wittes, R.E. and Ellenberg, S.S. 1985. Randomized phase II clinical trials. *Cancer Treatment Reports*, 69(12), 1375–1381.

Simon, R.M., Steinberg, S.M., Hamilton, M., Hildesheim, A., Khleif, S., Kwak, L.W., Mackall, C.L., Schlom, J., Topalian, S.L. and Berzofsky, J.A. 2001. Clinical trial designs for the early clinical development of therapeutic cancer vaccines. *Journal of Clinical Oncology*, 19(6), 1848–1854.

Slamon, D.J., Leyland-Jones, B., Shak, S., Fuchs, H., Paton, V., Bajamonde, A., Fleming, T., Eiermann, W., Wolter, J., Pegram, M., Baselga, J. and Norton, L. 2001. Use of chemotherapy plus a monoclonal antibody against HER2 for metastatic breast cancer that overexpresses HER2. *New England Journal of Medicine*, 344(11), 783–792.

Smith, M.R., Kabbinavar, F., Saad, F., Hussain, A., Gittelman, M.C., Bilhartz, D.L., Wynne, C., Murray, R., Zinner, N.R., Schulman, C., Linnartz, R., Zheng, M., Goessl, C., Hei, Y.J., Small, E.J., Cook, R. and Higano, C.S. 2005. Natural history of rising serum prostate-specific antigen in men with castrate nonmetastatic prostate cancer. *Journal of Clinical Oncology*, 23(13), 2918–2925.

Sobrero, A.F., Maurel, J., Fehrenbacher, L., Scheithauer, W., Abubakr, Y.A., Lutz, M.P., Vega-Villegas, M.E., Eng, C., Steinhauer, E.U., Prausova, J., Lenz, H.J., Borg, C., Middleton, G., Kröning, H., Luppi, G., Kisker, O., Zubel, A., Langer, C., Kopit, J. and Burris, H.A. 2008. EPIC: phase III trial of cetuximab plus irinotecan after fluoropyrimidine and oxaliplatin failure in patients with metastatic colorectal cancer. *Journal of Clinical Oncology*, 26(14), 2311–2319.

Stadler, W. 2002. New trial designs to assess antitumor and antiproliferative agents in prostate cancer. *Investigational New Drugs*, 20(2), 201–208.

Stadler, W.M. 2007. The randomized discontinuation trial: a phase II design to assess growth-inhibitory agents. *Molecular Cancer Therapeutics*, 6(4), 1180–1185.

Stallard, N. and Cockey, L. 2008. Two-stage designs for phase II cancer trials with ordinal responses. *Contemporary Clinical Trials*, 29(6), 896–904.

Stallard, N. and Todd, S. 2003. Sequential designs for phase III clinical trials incorporating treatment selection. *Statistics in Medicine*, 22(5), 689–703.

Steinberg, S.M. and Venzon, D.J. 2002. Early selection in a randomized phase II clinical trial. *Statistics in Medicine*, 21(12), 1711–1726.

Stone, A., Wheeler, C. and Barge, A. 2007a. Improving the design of phase II trials of cytostatic anticancer agents. *Contemporary Clinical Trials*, 28(2), 138–145.

Stone, A., Wheeler, C., Carroll, K. and Barge, A. 2007b. Optimizing randomized phase II trials assessing tumor progression. *Contemporary Clinical Trials*, 28(2), 146–152.

Storer, B.E. 1990. A sequential phase II/III trial for binary outcomes. *Statistics in Medicine*, 9(3), 229–235.

Storer, B.E. 1992. A class of phase II designs with three possible outcomes. *Biometrics*, 48(1), 55–60.

Sun, L.Z., Chen, C. and Patel, K. 2009. Optimal two-stage randomized multinomial designs for phase II oncology trials. *Journal of Biopharmaceutical Statistics*, 19(3), 485–493.

Sylvester, R.J. 1988. A Bayesian approach to the design of phase II clinical trials. *Biometrics*, 44(3), 823–836.

Sylvester, R.J. and Staquet, M.J. 1980. Design of phase II clinical trials in cancer using decision theory. *Cancer Treatment Reports*, 64(2–3), 519–524.

Tan, M. and Xiong, X. 1996. Continuous and group sequential conditional probability ratio tests for phase II clinical trials. *Statistics in Medicine*, 15(19), 2037–2051.

Tan, S.B. and Machin, D. 2002. Bayesian two-stage designs for phase II clinical trials. *Statistics in Medicine*, 21(14), 1991–2012.

Tang, H., Foster, N.R., Grothey, A., Ansell, S.M., Goldberg, R.M. and Sargent, D.J. 2010. Comparison of error rates in single-arm versus randomized phase II cancer clinical trials. *Journal of Clinical Oncology*, 28(11), 1936–1941.

Taylor, J.M., Braun, T.M. and Li, Z. 2006. Comparing an experimental agent to a standard agent: relative merits of a one-arm or randomized two-arm phase II design. *Clinical Trials*, 3(4), 335–348.

Thall, P.F. and Cheng, S.C. 1999. Treatment comparisons based on two-dimensional safety and efficacy alternatives in oncology trials. *Biometrics*, 55(3), 746–753.

Thall, P.F. and Cheng, S.C. 2001. Optimal two-stage designs for clinical trials based on safety and efficacy. *Statistics in Medicine*, 20(7), 1023–1032.

Thall, P.F. and Estey, E.H. 1993. A Bayesian strategy for screening cancer treatments prior to phase II clinical evaluation. *Statistics in Medicine*, 12(13), 1197–1211.

Thall, P.F., Millikan, R.E. and Sung, H.G. 2000. Evaluating multiple treatment courses in clinical trials. *Statistics in Medicine*, 19(8), 1011–1028.

Thall, P.F. and Simon, R. 1990. Incorporating historical control data in planning phase II clinical trials. *Statistics in Medicine*, 9(3), 215–228.

Thall, P.F. and Simon, R. 1994a. A Bayesian approach to establishing sample size and monitoring criteria for phase II clinical trials. *Controlled Clinical Trials*, 15(6), 463–481.

Thall, P.F. and Simon, R. 1994b. Practical Bayesian guidelines for phase IIB clinical trials. *Biometrics*, 50(2), 337–349.

Thall, P.F., Simon, R. and Estey, E.H. 1995. Bayesian sequential monitoring designs for single-arm clinical trials with multiple outcomes. *Statistics in Medicine*, 14, 357–379.

Thall, P.F., Simon, R.M. and Estey, E.H. 1996. New statistical strategy for monitoring safety and efficacy in single-arm clinical trials. *Journal of Clinical Oncology*, 14(1), 296–303.

Thall, P.F. and Sung, H.G. 1998. Some extensions and applications of a Bayesian strategy for monitoring multiple outcomes in clinical trials. *Statistics in Medicine*, 17(14), 1563–1580.

Thall, P.F., Wathen, J.K., Bekele, B.N., Champlin, R.E., Baker, L.H. and Benjamin, R.S. 2003. Hierarchical Bayesian approaches to phase II trials in diseases with multiple subtypes. *Statistics in Medicine*, 22(5), 763–780.

Thall, P.F., Wooten, L.H. and Tannir, N.M. 2005. Monitoring event times in early phase clinical trials: some practical issues. *Clinical Trials*, 2(6), 467–478.

Therasse, P. 2002. Measuring the clinical response. What does it mean? *European Journal of Cancer* 38(14), 1817–1823.

Tobias, J.S., Monson, K., Gupta, N., MacDougall, H., Glaholm, J., Hutchison, I., Kadalayil, L. and Hackshaw, A. 2010. Chemoradiotherapy for locally advanced head and neck cancer: 10-year follow-up of the UK Head and Neck (UKHAN1) trial. *The Lancet Oncology*, 11(1), 66–74.

Todd, S. and Stallard, N. 2005. A new clinical trial design combining phases 2 and 3: sequential designs with treatment selection and a change of endpoint. *Drug Information Journal*, 39(2), 109–118.

Tol, J., Koopman, M., Cats, A., Rodenburg, C.J., Creemers, G.J., Schrama, J.G., Erdkamp, F.L., Vos, A.H., van Groeningen, C.J., Sinnige, H.A., Richel, D.J., Voest, E.E., Dijkstra, J.R., Vink-Börger, M.E., Antonini, N.F., Mol, L., van Krieken, J.H., Dalesio, O. and Punt, C.J. 2009. Chemotherapy, bevacizumab, and cetuximab in metastatic colorectal cancer. *New England Journal of Medicine*, 360(6), 563–572.

Tournoux, C., De Rycke, Y., Medioni, J. and Asselain, B. 2007. Methods of joint evaluation of efficacy and toxicity in phase II clinical trials. *Contemporary Clinical Trials*, 28(4), 514–524.

Tournoux-Facon, C., De Rycke, Y. and Tubert-Bitter, P. 2011. Targeting population entering phase III trials: a new stratified adaptive phase II design. *Statistics in Medicine*, 30(8), 801–811.

Twombly, R. 2006. Criticism of tumor response criteria raises trial design questions. *Journal of the National Cancer Institute*, 98(4), 232–234.

U.S. Department of Health and Human Services, Food and Drug Administration, Center for Drug Evaluation and Research (CDER) 2013. *Guidance for Industry: Codevelopment of Two or More New Investigational Drugs for Use in Combination*. Final Draft June 2013. Available online at: http://www.fda.gov/Drugs/Guidance ComplianceRegulatoryInformation/Guidances/default.htm (accessed on 1 November 2013).

Van Cutsem, E., Kohne, C.H., Hitre, E., Zaluski, J., Chang Chien, C.R., Makhson, A., D'Haens, G., Pinter, T., Lim, R., Bodoky, G., Roh, J.K., Folprecht, G., Ruff, P., Stroh, C., Tejpar, S., Schlichting, M., Nippgen, J. and Rougier, P. 2009. Cetuximab and chemotherapy as initial treatment for metastatic colorectal cancer. *New England Journal of Medicine*, 360(14), 1408–1417.

van de Donk, N.W.C.J., Lokhorst, H.M., Dimopoulos, M., Cavo, M., Morgan, G., Einsele, H., Kropff, M., Schey, S., Avet-Loiseau, H., Ludwig, H., Goldschmidt, H., Sonneveld, P., Johnsen, H.E., Blade, J., San-Miguel, J.F. and Palumbo, A. 2011. Treatment of relapsed and refractory multiple myeloma in the era of novel agents. *Cancer Treatment Reviews*, 37(4), 266–283.

Van Glabbeke, M., Steward, W. and Armand, J.P. 2002. Non-randomised phase II trials of drug combinations: often meaningless, sometimes misleading. Are there alternative strategies? *European Journal of Cancer*, 38(5), 635–638.

Vickers, A.J. 2009. Phase II designs for anticancer botanicals and supplements. *Journal of the Society for Integrative Oncology*, 7(1), 35–40.

Vickers, A.J., Ballen, V. and Scher, H.I. 2007. Setting the bar in phase II trials: the use of historical data for determining 'go/no go' decision for definitive phase III testing. *Clinical Cancer Research*, 13(3), 972–976.

Von Hoff, D.D. 1998. There are no bad anticancer agents, only bad clinical trial designs – Twenty-First Richard and Hinda Rosenthal Foundation Award Lecture. *Clinical Cancer Research*, 4(5), 1079–1086.

Walker, I. and Newell, H. 2009. Do molecularly targeted agents in oncology have reduced attrition rates? *Nature Reviews Drug Discovery*, 8(1), 15–16.

Wang, J. 2006. An adaptive two-stage design with treatment selection using the conditional error function approach. *Biometrical Journal*, 48(4), 679–689.

Wang, L. and Cui, L. 2007. Seamless phase II/III combination study through response adaptive randomization. *Journal of Biopharmaceutical Statistics*, 17(6), 1177–1187.

Wang, Y.G., Leung, D.H., Li, M. and Tan, S.B. 2005. Bayesian designs with frequentist and Bayesian error rate considerations. *Statistical Methods in Medical Research*, 14(5), 445–456.

Wathen, J.K., Thall, P.F., Cook, J.D. and Estey, E.H. 2008. Accounting for patient heterogeneity in phase II clinical trials. *Statistics in Medicine*, 27(15), 2802–2815.

Weiss, G.B. and Hokanson, J.A. 1984. Advantages of integrated trials for performing multiple phase II studies. *Investigational New Drugs*, 2(4), 409–414.

Whitehead, J. 1985. Designing phase II studies in the context of a programme of clinical research. *Biometrics*, 41(2), 373–383.

Whitehead, J. 1986. Sample sizes for phase II and phase III clinical trials: an integrated approach. *Statistics in Medicine*, 5(5), 459–464.

Whitehead, J. 1997. *The Design and Analysis of Sequential Clinical Trials*, 2nd edn. John Wiley & Sons, Ltd, Chichester.

Whitehead, J. and Jaki, T. 2009. One- and two-stage design proposals for a phase II trial comparing three active treatments with control using an ordered categorical endpoint. *Statistics in Medicine*, 28(5), 828–847.

Whitehead, J., Valdes-Marquez, E. and Lissmats, A. 2009. A simple two-stage design for quantitative responses with application to a study in diabetic neuropathic pain. *Pharmaceutical Statistics*, 8(2), 125–135.

Wu, C. and Liu, A. 2007. An adaptive approach for bivariate phase II clinical trial designs. *Contemporary Clinical Trials*, 28(4), 482–486.

Wu, Y. and Shih, W.J. 2008. Approaches to handling data when a phase II trial deviates from the pre-specified Simon's two-stage design. *Statistics in Medicine*, 27(29), 6190–6208.

Ye, F. and Shyr, Y. 2007. Balanced two-stage designs for phase II clinical trials. *Clinical Trials*, 4(5), 514–524.

Yothers, G., Wieand, H.S. and Freireich, E.J. 2006. Pro/Con: randomization in phase II clinical trials. *Clinical Advances in Hematology and Oncology*, 4(10), 776–778.

Zee, B., Melnychuk, D., Dancey, J. and Eisenhauer, E. 1999. Multinomial phase II cancer trials incorporating response and early progression. *Journal of Biopharmaceutical Statistics*, 9(2), 351–363.

Index

A Practical Guide to Designing Phase II Trials in Oncology, First Edition.
Sarah R. Brown, Walter M. Gregory, Chris Twelves and Julia Brown.
© 2014 John Wiley & Sons, Ltd. Published 2014 by John Wiley & Sons, Ltd.

Statistics in Practice

Human and Biological Sciences

Berger – Selection Bias and Covariate Imbalances in Randomized Clinical Trials

Berger and Wong – An Introduction to Optimal Designs for Social and Biomedical Research

Brown, Gregory, Twelves and Brown – A Practical Guide to Designing Phase II Trials in Oncology

Brown and Prescott – Applied Mixed Models in Medicine, Second Edition

Carpenter and Kenward – Multiple Imputation and its Application

Carstensen – Comparing Clinical Measurement Methods

Chevret (Ed.) – Statistical Methods for Dose-Finding Experiments

Ellenberg, Fleming and DeMets – Data Monitoring Committees in Clinical Trials: A Practical Perspective

Hauschke, Steinijans and Pigeot – Bioequivalence Studies in Drug Development: Methods and Applications

Källén – Understanding Biostatistics

Lawson, Browne and Vidal Rodeiro – Disease Mapping with Win-BUGS and MLwiN

Lesaffre, Feine, Leroux and Declerck – Statistical and Methodological Aspects of Oral Health Research

Lui – Statistical Estimation of Epidemiological Risk

Marubini and Valsecchi – Analysing Survival Data from Clinical Trials and Observation Studies

Millar – Maximum Likelihood Estimation and Inference: With Examples in R, SAS and ADMB

Molenberghs and Kenward – Missing Data in Clinical Studies

Morton, Mengersen, Playford and Whitby – Statistical Methods for Hospital Monitoring with R

O'Hagan, Buck, Daneshkhah, Eiser, Garthwaite, Jenkinson, Oakley and Rakow – Uncertain Judgements: Eliciting Expert's Probabilities

O'Kelly and Ratitch – Clinical Trials with Missing Data: A Guide for Practitioners

Parmigiani – Modeling in Medical Decision Making: A Bayesian Approach

Pintilie – Competing Risks: A Practical Perspective

Senn – Cross-over Trials in Clinical Research, Second Edition

Senn – Statistical Issues in Drug Development, Second Edition

Spiegelhalter, Abrams and Myles – Bayesian Approaches to Clinical Trials and Health-Care Evaluation

Walters – Quality of Life Outcomes in Clinical Trials and Health-Care Evaluation

Welton, Sutton, Cooper and Ades – Evidence Synthesis for Decision Making in Healthcare

Whitehead – Design and Analysis of Sequential Clinical Trials, Revised Second Edition

Whitehead – Meta-Analysis of Controlled Clinical Trials

Willan and Briggs – Statistical Analysis of Cost Effectiveness Data

Winkel and Zhang – Statistical Development of Quality in Medicine

Earth and Environmental Sciences

Buck, Cavanagh and Litton – Bayesian Approach to Interpreting Archaeological Data
Chandler and Scott – Statistical Methods for Trend Detection and Analysis in the
    Environmental Statistics
Glasbey and Horgan – Image Analysis in the Biological Sciences
Haas – Improving Natural Resource Management: Ecological and Political Models
Haas – Introduction to Probability and Statistics for Ecosystem Managers
Helsel – Nondetects and Data Analysis: Statistics for Censored Environmental Data
Illian, Penttinen, Stoyan and Stoyan – Statistical Analysis and Modelling of Spatial Point
    Patterns
Mateu and Muller (Eds) – Spatio-Temporal Design: Advances in Efficient Data Acquisition
McBride – Using Statistical Methods for Water Quality Management
Webster and Oliver – Geostatistics for Environmental Scientists, Second Edition
Wymer (Ed.) – Statistical Framework for Recreational Water Quality Criteria and Monitoring

Industry, Commerce and Finance

Aitken – Statistics and the Evaluation of Evidence for Forensic Scientists, Second Edition
Balding – Weight-of-evidence for Forensic DNA Profiles
Brandimarte – Numerical Methods in Finance and Economics: A MATLAB-Based
    Introduction, Second Edition
Brandimarte and Zotteri – Introduction to Distribution Logistics
Chan – Simulation Techniques in Financial Risk Management
Coleman, Greenfield, Stewardson and Montgomery (Eds) – Statistical Practice in Business
    and Industry
Frisen (Ed.) – Financial Surveillance
Fung and Hu – Statistical DNA Forensics
Gusti Ngurah Agung – Time Series Data Analysis Using EViews
Jank and Shmueli (Ed.) – Statistical Methods in e-Commerce Research
Kenett (Ed.) – Operational Risk Management: A Practical Approach to Intelligent Data
    Analysis
Kenett (Ed.) – Modern Analysis of Customer Surveys: With Applications using R
Kenett and Zacks – Modern Industrial Statistics: With Applications in R, MINITAB and JMP,
    Second Edition
Kruger and Xie – Statistical Monitoring of Complex Multivariate Processes: With
    Applications in Industrial Process Control
Lehtonen and Pahkinen – Practical Methods for Design and Analysis of Complex Surveys,
    Second Edition
Ohser and Mücklich – Statistical Analysis of Microstructures in Materials Science
Pasiouras (Ed.) – Efficiency and Productivity Growth: Modelling in the Financial Services
    Industry
Pourret, Naim and Marcot (Eds) – Bayesian Networks: A Practical Guide to Applications
Ruggeri, Kenett and Faltin – Encyclopedia of Statistics and Reliability
Taroni, Aitken, Garbolino and Biedermann – Bayesian Networks and Probabilistic Inference
    in Forensic Science
Taroni, Bozza, Biedermann, Garbolino and Aitken – Data Analysis in Forensic Science

Printed and bound by CPI Group (UK) Ltd, Croydon, CR0 4YY

27/10/2024

14580349-0002
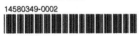